HEALTHY

0 POINT WEIGHT LOSS

COOKBOOK

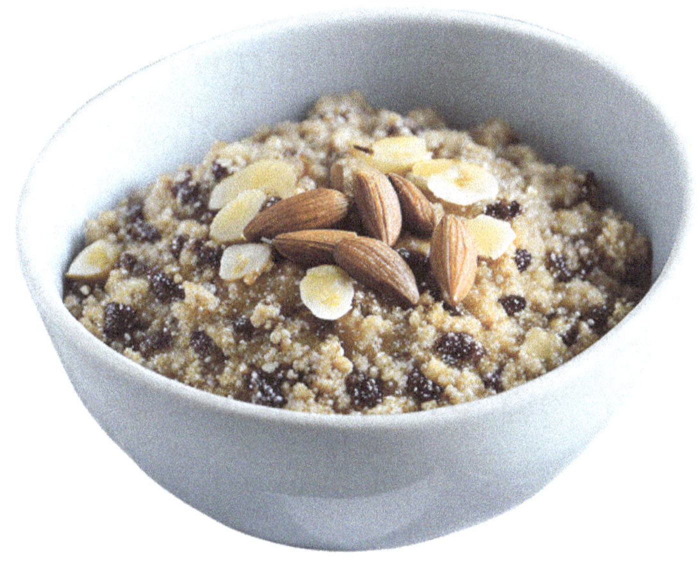

A 365 Days of Guilt-Free Delicious Recipes to enjoy on Every Meal. With Full-color pictures

Carla Campbell

All rights reserved Copyright @2024

No part of this publication may be reproduced, distributed, or transmitted in any means, including photocopying, Recording, or other electronic or mechanical methods, without the prior written permission of the publisher, except in the case of brief quotations Embodied in critical reviews and certain other noncommercial uses permitted by Copyright law.

Cover design by [Emily Thompson]

Illustrations by [David Martinez]

Edited by [Sarah Johnson]

Printed in the United States of America

The table of content

INTRODUCTION

In today's fast-paced world, the quest for effective and sustainable weight loss solutions has led many to explore various dietary approaches. Among these, zero-point weight loss has emerged as a powerful strategy for those seeking to shed pounds while maintaining a healthy, balanced diet. But what exactly does zero-point weight loss mean, and how can it transform your approach to eating and living?

The concept of zero-point weight reduction centers on eating foods naturally rich in nutrients and low in calories. These meals, often called "zero-point foods," may be consumed in large quantities without substantially changing the number of calories you consume each day. This idea is founded on the idea that not all calories are created equal and that some meals are better for you overall and for weight reduction than others.

Imagine living in a world where you can eat excellent, fulfilling meals without worrying about feeling hungry or missing out on anything. A society in which plenty replaces scarcity and shame gives way to nutrition. Zero-point weight loss offers a fun and sustainable approach to lose weight without compromising your enjoyment of food.

Benefits of Zero-Point Foods

Beyond only being suitable for those watching their calories, zero-point meals have several other advantages. They provide a comprehensive weight reduction method that prioritizes general health, fullness, and nutrition. The following are the main advantages of including zero-point items in your diet

1. Nutrient Density: Foods that score zero are usually high in essential minerals, vitamins, and antioxidants. These nutrients are essential for maintaining your body's processes, which include strengthening your immune system, promoting healthy skin, and lowering inflammation. You're improving your general health in addition to reducing weight by emphasizing nutrient-dense meals.

2. Satiety and Satisfaction: Controlling hunger and cravings is one of the most challenging aspects of weight reduction. Lean proteins, fruits, vegetables, and legumes are zero-point foods. Their high fiber and protein content makes them

feel fuller for longer. This makes it simpler to keep to your weight reduction strategy since you're less prone to overeat during meals or grab unhealthy snacks.

3. Flexibility and Freedom: Zero-point weight reduction allows flexibility and freedom, unlike restrictive diets that cut out whole food categories or need careful calorie tracking. You may indulge in an extensive range of meals without worrying about calories or portion sizes all the time. This method promotes attentive eating and a better connection with food.

4. Sustainable Weight Loss: Any weight reduction strategy must aim for sustainability. Fad diets and quick solutions often provide short-term effects and may even be detrimental. Zero-point weight loss encourages weight reduction that is more likely to be sustained over time since it is slow and continuous. Including healthy eating in your routine gives you the best chance of long-term success.

5. Better Digestive Health: Many foods with no points are fibre-rich, which is necessary for a healthy digestive system. In addition to facilitating digestion and preventing constipation, fibre supports a balanced gut flora. Maintaining a healthy digestive tract is essential for general health and may affect your energy and mood.

6. Enhanced Energy Levels: Consuming meals high in nutrients and low in points will help you feel more energized all day. Your body gets the energy it needs to perform at its best when you feed it healthful, natural foods. This may result in higher output, improved training, and an active lifestyle.

Starting a zero-point weight reduction program is about living a healthier, more energetic life rather than merely reducing weight. It's about enjoying the food you consume and feeling good about nourishing your body. Explore the world of zero-point recipes, and you'll find a wide variety of tasty, filling dishes that will help you achieve your weight reduction objectives and improve your general health—greetings from a new chapter of healthy food, optimal health, and living your best life.

How to Use This Book for Your Weight Loss Journey

Starting a weight reduction journey may be an exciting and challenging experience. This book is meant to serve as your all-in-one resource, offering you delectable zero-point recipes to make you feel good about every mouthful of your weight reduction journey. Here's how to get the most out of this book and guarantee a happy and successful journey

Step 1: Understanding the Basics

Spend time understanding the fundamentals of zero-point weight reduction before tackling the recipes. Learn about the kinds of meals regarded as zero-point and the reasons for their advantages for general health and weight reduction. You may optimize the benefits of the recipes in this book and make well-informed decisions with the support of this fundamental information.

Step 2: Setting Realistic Goals

Establishing attainable and reasonable objectives is essential for long-term success. Think about the goals you have for your weight reduction journey. Setting specific objectives can help you stay motivated and focused, whether you aim to lose weight, increase your energy, or change your diet. Recall that progress, not perfection, is the goal of this trip.

Step 3: Planning Your Meals

A crucial element of a successful weight reduction strategy is meal planning. Use this book to create a weekly food plan. Select a range of recipes from various departments to guarantee that your diet is well-balanced and full of all the necessary nutrients. If you plan beforehand, you'll save time and resist the urge to grab unhealthy items.

Step 4: Shopping for Ingredients

Once you've chosen your recipes, make a list of the items you'll need for your shopping list. Fresh, complete foods are often zero-point items, although they can require more regular supermarket shopping. Make buying fresh produce, lean meats, and other zero-point staples a top priority. Maintaining your food plan will be simpler if you have these items.

Step 5: Preparing Your Meals

One of the finest ways to take charge of your nutrition is to cook at home. Follow the recipes in this book to make tasty zero-point dinners. Vary the flavors and preparation methods to make your meals engaging and pleasurable. Remember that the idea is to prepare meals that you like eating rather than ones that seem forced.

Step 6: Listening to Your Body

Observe your body's reaction as you begin including zero-point meals in your diet. Note your feelings after eating certain meals and modify your diet plan appropriately. Since every individual's physique is unique, what suits one person may not suit another. Recognize when you are hungry and complete, and don't be scared to modify recipes to your tastes and preferences.

Step 7: Staying Consistent

The secret to reaching your weight reduction objectives is consistency. While the odd indulgence is OK, make every effort to follow your food plan. Experiment with the many recipes in this book to make your diet interesting and avoid boredom. Recall that this trip aims to develop long-term, healthy behaviours rather than quick cures.

Step 8: Tracking Your Progress

Record your progress throughout your weight reduction journey. You can use a notebook, an app, or even routine self-check-ins. Honor your accomplishments, no matter how little, and turn failures into teaching moments. Keeping track of your development can inspire and allow you to recognize your progress.

Lastly, remember to enjoy the trip. Losing weight is a journey, and it's important to celebrate the little victories you have along the road. Accept the healthier version of yourself and enjoy finding delicious, nourishing foods that fill you up. This book is meant to guide you through every stage, giving you the motivation and resources you need to succeed.

By following these steps and using this book as your guide, you'll be well on your way to achieving your weight loss goals with zero-point recipes. Here's to a healthier, happier you!

Chapter 1: What Are Zero-Point Foods?

Imagine living in a world where portion sizes and calorie counts don't matter, and you can eat anything. This is the secret to the success of zero-point meals. This idea has wholly changed healthy eating and weight reduction. However, what precisely are meals with 0 points, and why are they so unique?

Zero-point foods are foods that you can eat without worrying about how many calories they contain. Generally speaking, they are high in water content and fiber, low in calories, and rich in vital nutrients. These items are the cornerstone of a nutritious, well-balanced diet, enabling you to reach your weight reduction objectives while enjoying moderate quantities. Incorporating zero-point items into your diet provides a more flexible and sustainable approach than conventional dieting, sometimes requiring stringent limitations and thorough monitoring. These meals encourage long-lasting, better eating habits by enabling you to concentrate on the quality of your diet rather than simply the amount.

Nutritional Benefits

The remarkable nutritional profile of zero-point meals is what makes them beautiful. Consuming these meals gives your body the vital nutrients it needs to flourish and aid in weight reduction efforts. The following are a few of the fantastic nutritional advantages of zero-point foods:

1. Rich in Essential Vitamins and Minerals

Foods marked as zero points are often loaded with vital vitamins and minerals essential for good health. For example, fruits and vegetables are rich in potassium, magnesium, folate, and vitamins A, C, and K. These nutrients are essential for maintaining bone, cardiovascular, and immune system health as well as optimum bodily performance.

2. High in Fiber

One of the best qualities of zero-point meals is the high fiber content. Fiber is crucial for digestive health because it helps control bowel movements, avoids constipation, and supports a healthy gut microbiota. Additionally, by encouraging feelings of fullness and lowering total calorie consumption, fibre lowers cholesterol, helps maintain blood sugar levels, and helps with weight management.

3. Low in Calories and Fat

Naturally low in calories and fat, zero-point meals are an excellent option for losing weight. By including these items in your diet, you can make filling meals that won't impede your growth. Non-starchy veggies, such as peppers, spinach, and broccoli, have a high volume and few calories, so you may eat guilt-free in large quantities4. High Water Content
Many zero-point items, particularly fruits and vegetables, are rich in water. This promotes a sensation of fullness and keeps you hydrated. Cooling and filling foods, including cucumber, strawberries, and watermelon, are ideal for meals and snacks.

5. Lean Protein Sources

Skinless chicken breast, turkey, and several fish varieties are examples of lean proteins often included on the list of zero-point items. Protein is an essential macronutrient that promotes muscle development and repair, increases metabolism, and keeps you feeling full and content. Consuming lean protein may help you lose weight by maintaining lean muscle mass and encouraging fat loss.

6. High in Antioxidants

Antioxidants, which help shield your body from oxidative stress and inflammation, are abundant in zero-point meals. For instance, berries are a great source of antioxidants like vitamin C and flavonoids that boost immunity and may lower the risk of chronic illnesses. Consuming a diet high in foods high in antioxidants can improve your general health and wellbeing.

Real-Life Examples of Zero-Point Foods

Here are some typical zero-point meals you can start including in your diet. These foods are not only tasty but also a great source of vital nutrients that promote your general health. Here are a few popular categories of meals that have no points that you may freely indulge in:

Fruits

Fruits are the natural sweetener of nature, packed full of vitamins, minerals, and antioxidants. Their high fibre and high water content make you feel satiated and full. Among the well-liked zero-point fruits are:

- Apples: An excellent snack and a healthy source of nutritional fibre, apples are crisp and delicious.
- Bananas: Rich in potassium, bananas are an excellent rapid energy source.
 Berries: High in vitamins and antioxidants, including raspberries, blackberries, blueberries, and strawberries.
- Oranges: A tasty and hydrating snack, oranges are high in vitamin C.
- Grapes: Rich in vitamins and antioxidants, grapes are a convenient snack to take on the move.
- Watermelon: Watermelon is low in calories and hydrating due to its high water content.

Vegetables

As they are low in calories and packed with various nutrients, vegetables are the foundation of every balanced diet. Due to their versatility, they may be included in almost every meal. Common veggies with 0 points are:
- Leafy Greens: Rich in vitamins and minerals, lettuce, kale, and spinach are all excellent choices.
- Broccoli: Packed in fiber, vitamins C and K, and folate, broccoli is a cruciferous vegetable.
- Carrots: Packed in beta-carotene, carrots make a delicious snack or addition to meals.
- Bell Peppers: These colorful veggies are abundant in vitamin C and antioxidants.
- Zucchini: An excellent complement to meals, zucchini is low in calories and works well in various cuisines.

- Tomatoes: Rich in vitamins C and K, tomatoes taste tremendous both cooked and raw.

Lean Proteins

- In addition to keeping you fuller for longer, protein is necessary for the synthesis and repair of tissues. Lean protein consumption may improve general health and muscle maintenance. Typical lean zer-point proteins are as follows:
- Skinless Chicken Breast: This versatile protein source is excellent for various dishes.
- Turkey Breast: Another nutrient-dense, adaptable lean protein choice.
- Tofu: A versatile plant-based protein that takes on flavor well in various cooking applications.
- Lentils and Beans: Rich in fibre and protein, lentils and beans are a great source of plant-based protein.
- Fish: Omega3 fatty acids and protein are abundant in several fish species, including tilapia and salmon.

Dairy

Some dairy products that are minimal in fat and provide calcium and other necessary elements without packing on the calories may also be categorized as zero-point meals. Typical dairy alternatives with 0 points are:

- Nonfat Plain Yoghurt: This adaptable yoghurt may be used in savoury and sweet recipes. It is a beautiful source of probiotics and calcium.
- Cottage Cheese with Low Fat: Cottage cheese is a satisfying and healthy choice since it is high in calcium and protein.

Combining Foods with Zero Points

One of their finest qualities is the ease with which zero-point items may be mixed to make delicious, filling meals. As an illustration:
Fruit Salad: Combine several low-point fruits to create an excellent, nutrient-dense snack or dessert.

- Veggie StirFry: Sauté a variety of zero-point veggies together with tofu to make a fast and nutritious supper.

- Chicken Salad: For a filling lunch, toss lean chicken breast with bell peppers, leafy greens, and a mild vinaigrette.

The Bond Emotionally

When you start including zero-point items in your regular meals, you may notice a significant change in your eating patterns and general perspective on food. Realizing you can eat a wide range of tasty, healthful meals without worrying about constantly monitoring your calorie intake is a liberating feeling. This feeling of freedom is inspiring and energizing, supporting you in sticking with your weight reduction plan.
Additionally, zero point meals will support your steady weight reduction, better digestion, and enhanced energy levels—all of which you'll see and feel in your body. You'll start to enjoy eating healthily, look forward to meals, and experiment with new dishes.

In the next few chapters, we'll explore a veritable gold mine of delicious and healthful zero point meals. There are many alternatives to fit every taste and occasion, from filling meals to appetizing snacks and robust breakfasts. Each dish is carefully created with healthy ingredients that will satisfy your senses and feed your body.

Its time to cook

CHAPTER TWO

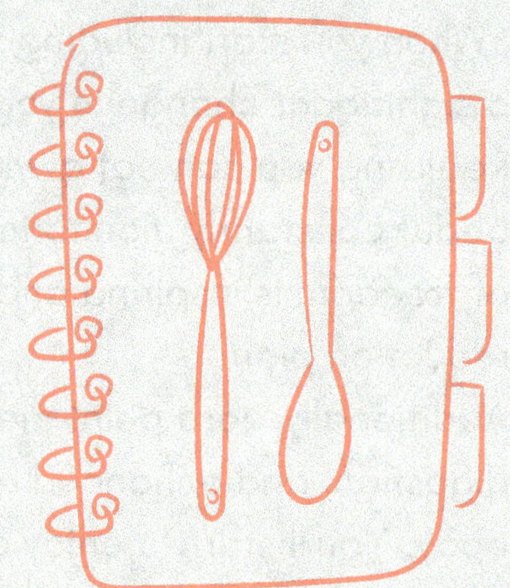

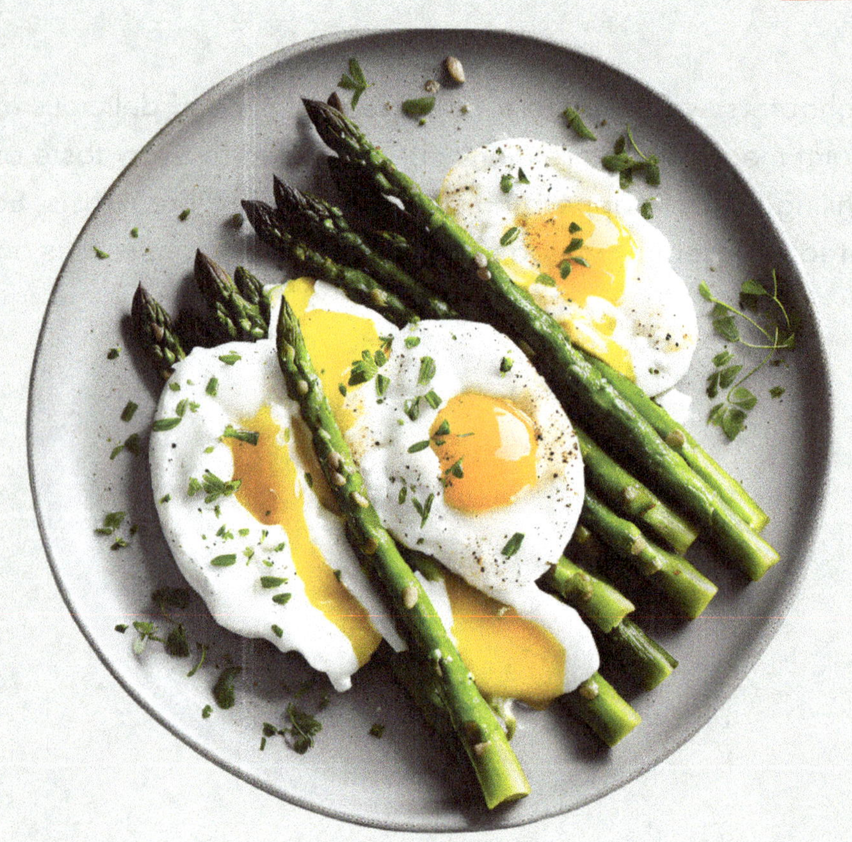

Breakfast Recipes

Start your day with this delightful Banana and Peanut Butter Toast! This recipe combines the creamy goodness of peanut butter with the natural sweetness of banana on a crispy toast. It's a quick, nutritious, and satisfying breakfast that feels like a treat but is guiltfree.

Banana and Peanut Butter Toast

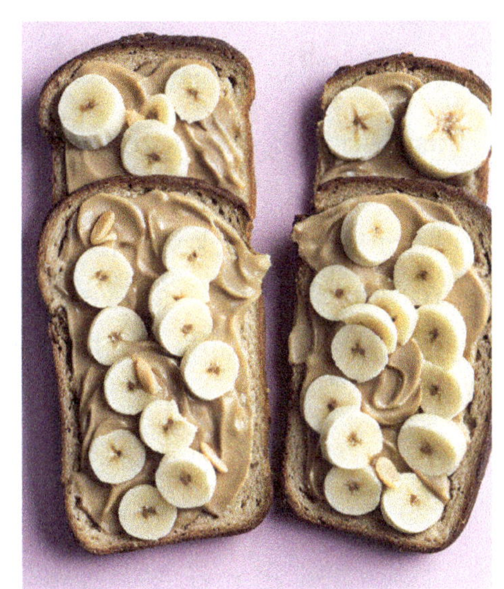

Preparation Time

Total: 5 minutes

Nutrition (per serving)

Calories: 210
Protein: 6g
Carbohydrates: 34g
Fiber: 5g
Fat: 8g

ingredients

- 1 slice of whole grain bread
- 1 tablespoon natural peanut butter (no added sugar)
- 1 small banana, sliced
- A pinch of cinnamon (optional)

Instructions

1. Toast the slice of whole grain bread until golden brown and crispy.
2. Spread the natural peanut butter evenly over the warm toast.
3. Arrange the banana slices on top of the peanut butter.
4. Sprinkle a pinch of cinnamon on top, if desired.
5. Serve immediately and enjoy!

About the recipe

This Vegetable Frittata is a colorful, delicious, and nutritious way to start your day or enjoy a light lunch. Packed with fresh veggies and proteinrich eggs, it's a versatile dish that's as healthy as it is tasty.

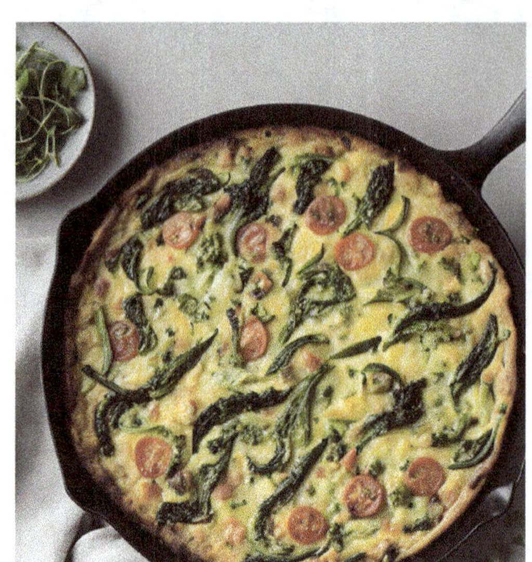

Vegetable Frittata

Preparation Time

Total: 30 minutes

Nutrition (per serving)

Calories: 140
Protein: 12g
Carbohydrates: 6g
Fiber: 2g
Fat: 8g

ingredients

- Cooking spray
- 1 small onion, diced
- 1 bell pepper, diced
- 1 cup spinach
- 6 eggs
- Salt and pepper to taste
- 1/4 cup lowfat milk (optional)

Instructions

1. Preheat your oven to 375°F (190°C).
2. Spray a nonstick skillet with cooking spray and heat over medium heat.
3. Add the onion and bell pepper to the skillet, cooking until they soften, about 5 minutes.
4. Add the spinach and cook until wilted, about 2 minutes.
5. In a bowl, beat the eggs with salt, pepper, and milk (if using).
6. Pour the egg mixture over the vegetables in the skillet.
7. Transfer the skillet to the preheated oven and bake until the frittata is set and golden about 1520 minutes.
8. Let it cool slightly before slicing and serving.

Kickstart your morning with this hearty Sweet Potato and Black Bean Breakfast Burrito. It's a flavorful, filling, and nutritious breakfast option for onthego mornings or a leisurely weekend brunch

Sweet Potato and Black Bean Breakfast Burrito

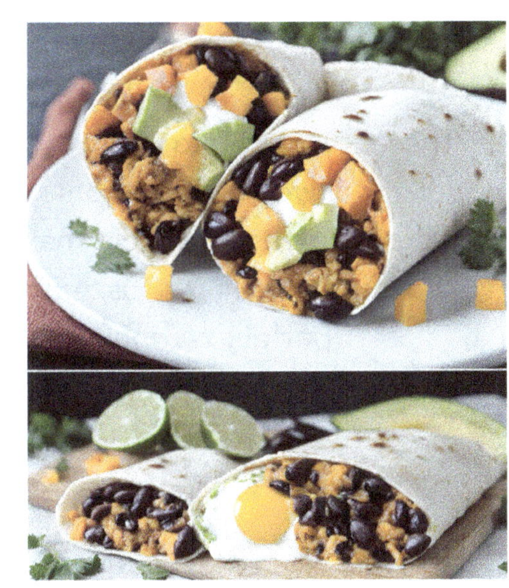

Preparation Time

Total: 25 minutes

Nutrition (per serving)

Calories: 250
Protein: 12g
Carbohydrates: 42g
Fiber: 8g
Fat: 6g

ingredients

- 1 medium sweet potato, peeled and diced
- 1/2 cup black beans, drained and rinsed
- 1 small onion, diced
- 1 bell pepper, diced
- 2 eggs
- 2 whole wheat tortillas
- Cooking spray
- Salt and pepper to taste

Instructions

1. Spray a skillet with cooking spray and heat over medium heat.

2. Add the sweet potato and cook until it softens, about 10 minutes.

3. Add the onion and bell pepper, cooking until all vegetables are tender, about five more minutes.

4. Stir in the black beans and cook until heated, about 2 minutes.

5. In another skillet, scramble the eggs until just set, about 3 minutes.

6. Warm the tortillas in the microwave or skillet for about 30 seconds.

7. Fill each tortilla with the sweet potato mixture and scrambled eggs, then roll into burritos.

8. Serve immediately or wrap in foil for a convenient onthego option.

About the recipe

These Zucchini and Carrot Muffins are a delightful way to sneak some veggies into your breakfast or snack. They are moist, flavorful, and nutritious, making them a perfect zeropoint treat.

Zucchini and Carrot Muffin

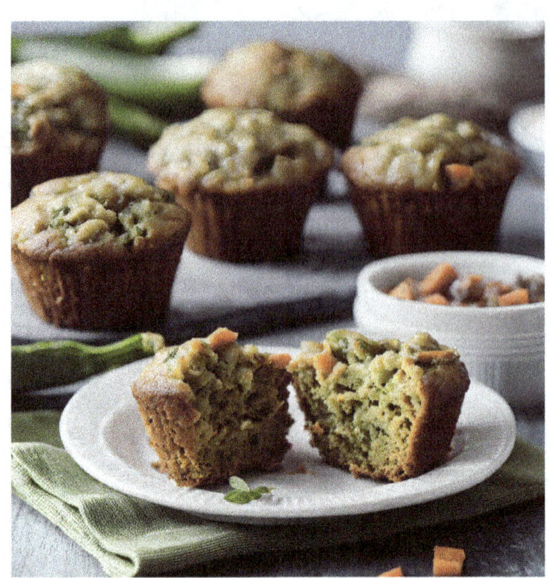

Preparation Time

Total: 35 minutes

Nutrition (per serving)

Calories: 100
Protein: 3g
Carbohydrates: 20g
Fiber: 3g
Fat: 2g

ingredients

- 1 cup grated zucchini
- 1 cup grated carrot
- 1 cup whole wheat flour
- 1/2 cup unsweetened applesauce
- 2 eggs
- 1 teaspoon baking powder
- 1/2 teaspoon baking soda
- 1 teaspoon cinnamon
- 1/2 teaspoon salt
- Cooking spray

Instructions

1. Preheat your oven to 350°F (175°C) and spray a muffin tin with cooking spray.
2. combine the grated zucchini, carrot, and applesauce in a large bowl.
3. Add the eggs and mix well.
4. whisk together the flour, baking powder, baking soda, cinnamon, and salt in a separate bowl.
5. Gradually add the dry ingredients to the wet ingredients, mixing until combined.
6. Divide the batter evenly among the muffin cups.
7. Bake for 2025 minutes or until a toothpick inserted into the center comes clean.
8. Allow to cool before serving.

About the recipe

This Tomato and Basil Bruschetta is a refreshing and tasty appetizer or snack. The combination of ripe tomatoes, fresh basil, and a hint of garlic on toasted bread is irresistible and perfect for any time of the day.

Tomato and Basil Bruschetta

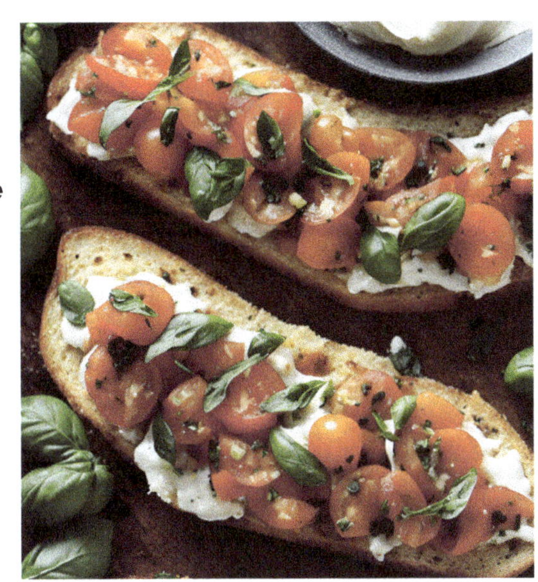

Preparation Time

Total: 15 minutes

Nutrition (per serving)

Calories: 80
Protein: 2g
Carbohydrates: 14g
Fiber: 1g
Fat: 1g

ingredients

- 4 ripe tomatoes, diced
- 1/4 cup fresh basil, chopped
- 2 cloves garlic, minced
- 1 tablespoon balsamic vinegar
- Salt and pepper to taste
- 1 baguette, sliced
- Cooking spray

Instructions

1. Preheat your oven to 400°F (200°C).

2. combine the diced tomatoes, basil, garlic, balsamic vinegar, salt, and pepper in a bowl.

3. Spray the baguette slices with cooking spray and place them on a baking sheet.

4. Toast the baguette slices in the oven until golden brown, about 57 minutes.

5. Spoon the tomato mixture onto the toasted baguette slices.

6. Serve immediately and enjoy the burst of fresh flavors.

Start your day with this luxurious Smoked Salmon and Avocado Bagel! It's a delightful combination of creamy avocado and rich smoked salmon on a wholegrain bagel, perfect for a nutritious and satisfying breakfast that feels like a treat.

Smoked Salmon and Avocado Bagel

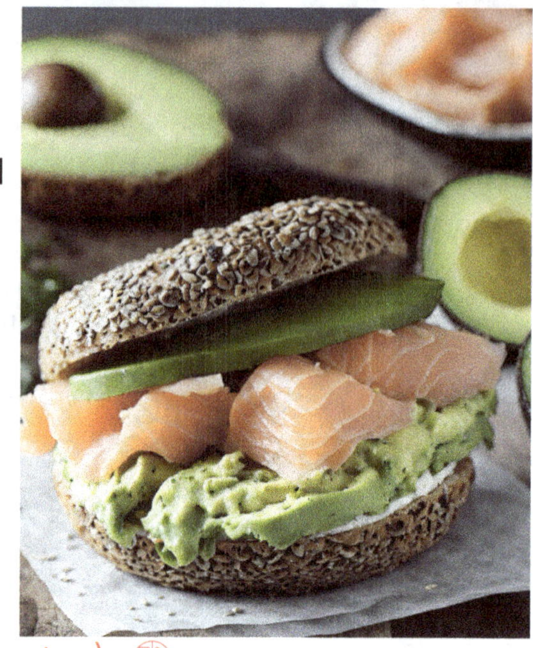

Preparation Time

Total: 10 minutes

Nutrition (per serving)

Calories: 290
Protein: 15g
Carbohydrates: 32g
Fiber: 8g
Fat: 14g

ingredients

- 1 whole grain bagel, sliced
- 1/2 ripe avocado, mashed
- 2 oz smoked salmon
- A squeeze of lemon juice
- A pinch of salt and pepper
- Fresh dill for garnish (optional)

Instructions

1. Toast the wholegrain bagel slices until golden brown.
2. Spread the mashed avocado evenly over each bagel half.
3. Top with smoked salmon slices.
4. Squeeze some lemon juice over the salmon and sprinkle with salt and pepper.
5. Garnish with fresh dill if desired.
6. Serve immediately and enjoy the delicious combination of flavors!

About the recipe

Overnight oats are a lifesaver for busy mornings, and this Raspberry and Chia version is delicious and nutritious. Prep it the night before and wake up to a readytoeat breakfast bursting with flavor and health benefits.

Overnight Oats with Raspberry and Chia

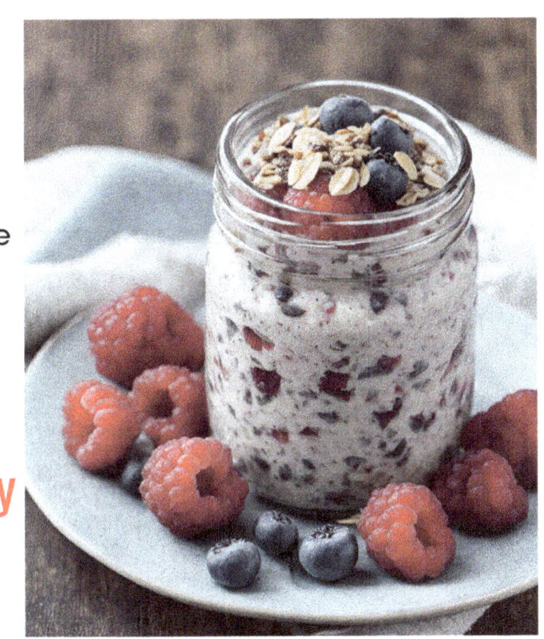

Preparation Time

Total: 5 minutes

Nutrition (per serving)

Calories: 220
Protein: 6g
Carbohydrates: 36g
Fiber: 10g
Fat: 7g

ingredients

- 1/2 cup rolled oats
- 1/2 cup unsweetened almond milk
- 1/2 cup fresh raspberries
- 1 tablespoon chia seeds
- 1 teaspoon honey (optional)
- A pinch of cinnamon

Instructions

1. combine the rolled oats, almond milk, chia seeds, and cinnamon in a jar or bowl.

2. Stir in the fresh raspberries, crushing a few to release their juice.

3. If desired, add a teaspoon of honey for extra sweetness.

4. Cover and refrigerate overnight.

5. In the morning, stir it well and enjoy it directly from the jar or transfer it to a bowl.

About the recipe

Elevate your scrambled eggs with this Mushroom and Spinach version. It's a simple, quick, and nutrientpacked breakfast that will keep you full and satisfied until lunchtime. Plus, it's a delicious way to start your day!

Mushroom and Spinach Scrambled Eggs

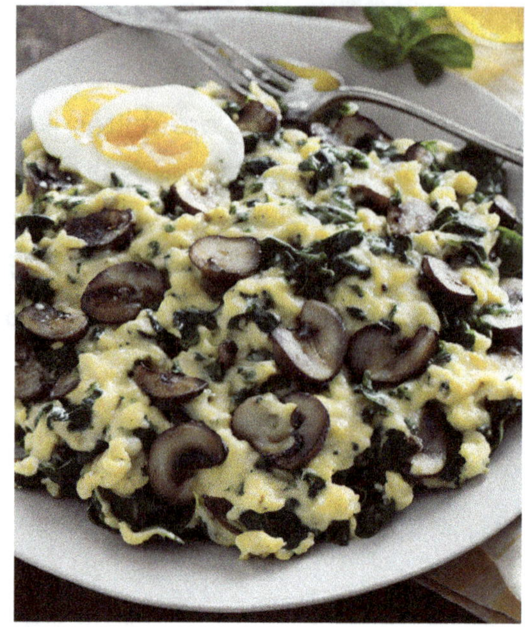

Preparation Time

Total: 10 minutes

Nutrition (per serving)

Calories: 180
Protein: 15g
Carbohydrates: 5g
Fiber: 2g
Fat: 12g

ingredients

- Cooking spray
- 1 cup sliced mushrooms
- 1 cup fresh spinach
- 3 eggs
- Salt and pepper to taste

Instructions

1. Spray a nonstick skillet with cooking spray and heat over medium heat.

2. Add the mushrooms and cook until they soften, about 5 minutes.

3. Add the spinach and cook until wilted, about 2 minutes.

4. whisk the eggs with a pinch of salt and pepper in a bowl.

5. Pour the eggs into the skillet and cook, stirring gently, until they are just set, about 34 minutes.

6. Serve immediately for a warm, savory breakfast.

About the recipe

Indulge in a breakfast classic with a healthy twist! These Whole Grain Waffles with Fresh Strawberries are delicious and packed with fibre and nutrients, making them a guiltfree treat for any morning.

Whole Grain Waffles with Fresh Strawberries

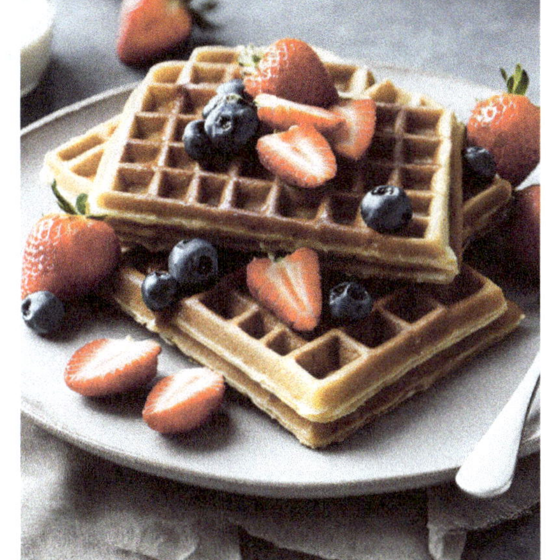

Preparation Time

Total: 20 minutes

Nutrition (per serving)

Calories: 250
Protein: 8g
Carbohydrates: 45g
Fiber: 8g
Fat: 5g

ingredients

- 1 cup whole grain flour
- 1 teaspoon baking powder
- 1/4 teaspoon salt
- 1 egg
- 1 cup unsweetened almond milk
- 1 tablespoon honey
- 1 cup fresh strawberries, sliced

Instructions

1. Preheat your waffle iron.

2. whisk the wholegrain flour, baking powder, and salt in a bowl.

3. In another bowl, beat the egg and add almond milk and honey.

4. Combine the wet and dry ingredients, mixing until just combined.

5. Pour the batter into the preheated waffle iron and cook according to the manufacturer's instructions until golden brown.

6. Top with fresh strawberries and serve immediately.

About the recipe

This Mixed Berry and Chia Smoothie is a refreshing, nutrientpacked way to start your day or enjoy as a midday snack. It's bursting with berry flavours, and the added chia seeds provide a great source of fibre and omega3s.

Mixed Berry and Chia Smoothie

Preparation Time

Total: 5 minutes

Nutrition (per serving)

Calories: 150
Protein: 3g
Carbohydrates: 30g
Fiber: 10g
Fat: 4g

ingredients

- 1 cup mixed berries (strawberries, blueberries, raspberries)
- 1 cup unsweetened almond milk
- 1 tablespoon chia seeds
- 1 teaspoon honey (optional)
- A few ice cubes

Instructions

1. Combine all the ingredients in a blender.
2. Blend until smooth.
3. Pour into a glass and enjoy immediately.

This Spinach and Feta Omelet is a delightful, proteinpacked breakfast that's both healthy and delicious. The combination of fresh spinach and tangy feta cheese makes for a savoury start to your day

Spinach and Feta Omelet

Preparation Time

Total: 10 minutes

Nutrition (per serving)

Calories: 200
Protein: 14g
Carbohydrates: 3g
Fiber: 1g
Fat: 15g

ingredients

- Cooking spray
- 1 cup fresh spinach
- 2 eggs
- 1/4 cup feta cheese, crumbled
- Salt and pepper to taste

Instructions

1. Spray a nonstick skillet with cooking spray and heat over medium heat.

2. Add the spinach and cook until wilted, about 2 minutes.

3. Whisk the eggs with a pinch of salt and pepper in a bowl.

4. Pour the eggs over the spinach in the skillet.

5. Cook until the eggs are set, then sprinkle the feta cheese on half the omelette.

6. Fold the omelette in half and cook for another minute until the cheese is slightly melted.

7. Serve immediately for a warm, savoury breakfast.

Kickstart your morning with this Avocado and Egg Breakfast Wrap! It's a delicious, proteinpacked wrap that combines creamy avocado with perfectly scrambled eggs, all wrapped up in a whole wheat tortilla.

Avocado and Egg Breakfast Wrap

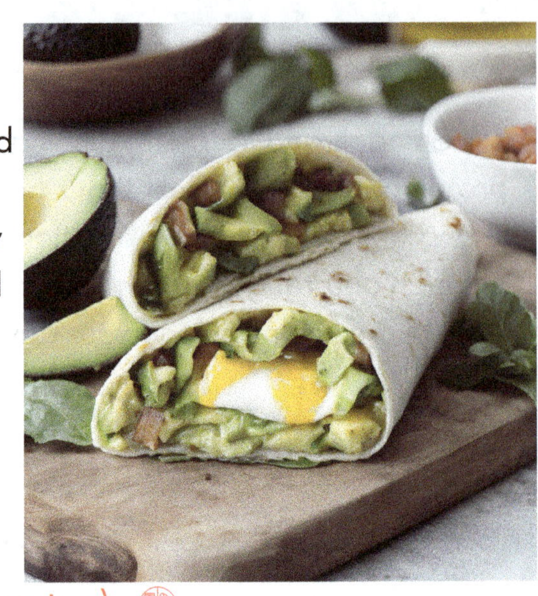

Preparation Time

Total: 10 minutes

Nutrition (per serving)

Calories: 320
Protein: 14g
Carbohydrates: 28g
Fiber: 10g
Fat: 18g

ingredients

- 1 whole wheat tortilla
- 1/2 ripe avocado, sliced
- 2 eggs
- A handful of baby spinach
- Salt and pepper to taste
- Cooking spray

Instructions

1. Spray a nonstick skillet with cooking spray and heat over medium heat.

2. Crack the eggs into a bowl, add a pinch of salt and pepper, and whisk until well blended.

3. Pour the eggs into the skillet and scramble until set about 34 minutes.

4. Warm the tortilla in the microwave or skillet for 30 seconds.

5. Place the scrambled eggs in the centre of the tortilla.

6. Top with sliced avocado and baby spinach.

7. Roll up the tortilla to form a wrap, securing it with a toothpick if necessary.

8. Serve immediately and enjoy!

About the recipe

This Greek Yogurt with Honey and Walnuts combines creamy, tangy yoghurt, sweet honey, and crunchy walnuts. It's a simple yet satisfying breakfast or snack that's both nutritious and delicious.

Greek Yogurt with Honey and Walnuts

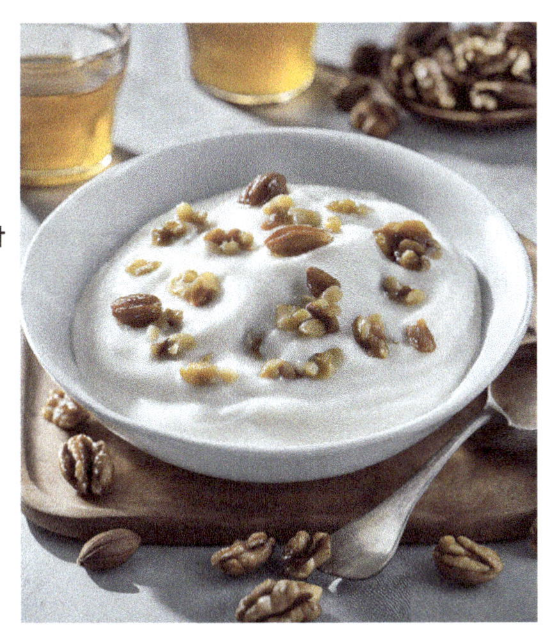

Preparation Time

Total: 5 minutes

Nutrition (per serving)

Calories: 200
Protein: 15g
Carbohydrates: 18g
Fiber: 2g
Fat: 8g

ingredients

- 1 cup plain Greek yoghurt
- 1 tablespoon honey
- 2 tablespoons chopped walnuts

Instructions

1. Spoon the Greek yoghurt into a bowl.

2. Drizzle the honey over the yoghurt.

3. Sprinkle the chopped walnuts on top.

4. Serve immediately and enjoy the perfect blend of flavours and textures.

About the recipe

These Almond Flour Pancakes with Blueberries are a healthy twist on a breakfast favourite. Light, fluffy, and bursting with juicy blueberries, these pancakes are glutenfree, low in carbs, and delicious.

Almond Flour Pancakes with Blueberries

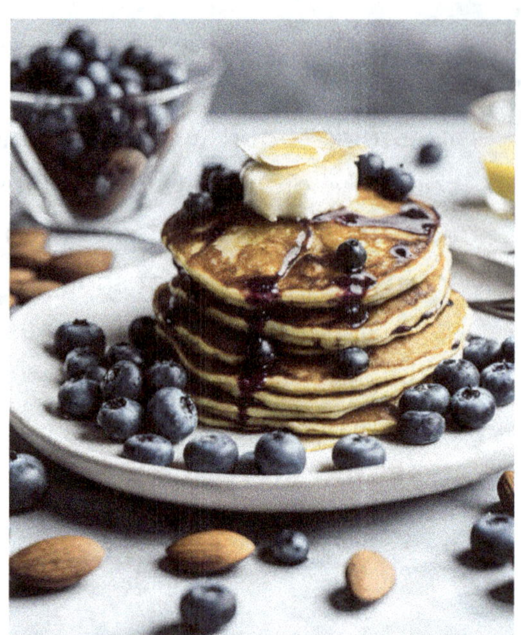

Preparation Time

Total: 15 minutes

Nutrition (per serving)

Calories: 220
Protein: 10g
Carbohydrates: 14g
Fiber: 4g
Fat: 14g

ingredients

- 1 cup almond flour
- 2 eggs
- 1/4 cup unsweetened almond milk
- 1 teaspoon baking powder
- 1 teaspoon vanilla extract
- 1/2 cup fresh blueberries
- Cooking spray

Instructions

1. whisk the almond flour, baking powder, eggs, almond milk, and vanilla extract until smooth.

2. Gently fold in the fresh blueberries.

3. Spray a nonstick skillet with cooking spray and heat over medium heat.

4. Pour 1/4 cup of the batter onto the skillet for each pancake.

5. Cook until bubbles form on the surface, then flip and cook until golden brown on both sides, about 23 minutes per side.

6. Serve warm and enjoy with extra blueberries on top if desired.

About the recipe

This Quinoa Breakfast Bowl with Mixed Fruit is a powerpacked way to start your day. With proteinrich quinoa and various fresh fruits, this bowl is not only colourful but also incredibly nutritious and filling.

Quinoa Breakfast Bowl with Mixed Fruit

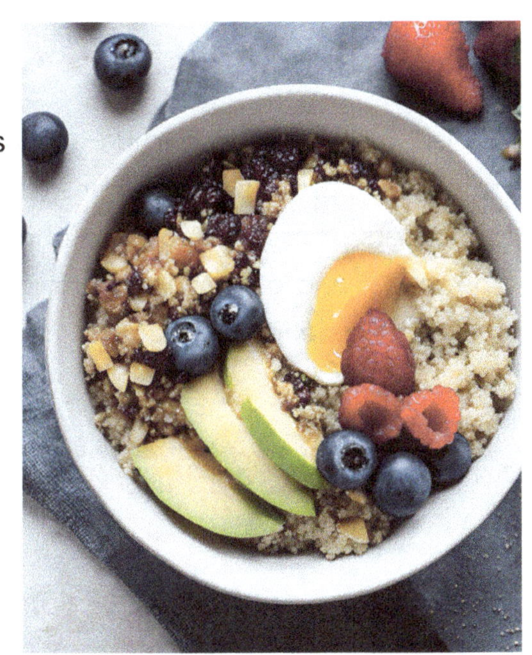

Preparation Time

Total: 10 minutes

Nutrition (per serving)

Calories: 250
Protein: 6g
Carbohydrates: 52g
Fiber: 8g
Fat: 4g

ingredients

- 1/2 cup cooked quinoa
- 1/2 cup fresh strawberries, sliced
- 1/2 cup fresh blueberries
- 1 small banana, sliced
- 1 tablespoon chia seeds
- 1 tablespoon honey (optional)

Instructions

1. Cook the quinoa according to package instructions and let it cool slightly.

2. combine the cooked quinoa with the sliced strawberries, blueberries, and banana in a bowl.

3. Sprinkle with chia seeds and drizzle with honey if desired.

4. Serve immediately and enjoy the fresh, vibrant flavours.

About the recipe

This Cottage Cheese and Peach Parfait is a refreshing, protein packed breakfast or snack. Layers of creamy cottage cheese, juicy peaches, and a sprinkle of granola make this parfait a delightful, healthy, and satisfying treat.

Cottage Cheese and Peach Parfait

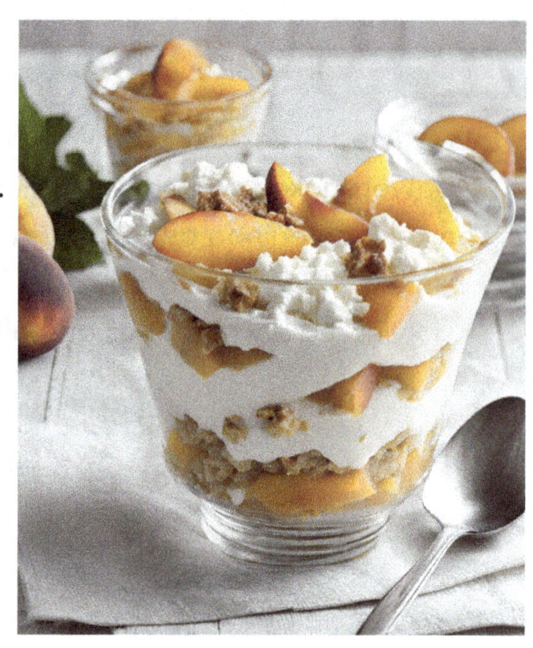

Preparation Time

Total: 5 minutes

Nutrition (per serving)

Calories: 180
Protein: 15g
Carbohydrates: 18g
Fiber: 2g
Fat: 5g

ingredients

- 1 cup lowfat cottage cheese
- 1 ripe peach, sliced
- 2 tablespoons granola
- A drizzle of honey (optional)

Instructions

1. layer half of the cottage cheese in a glass or bowl.

2. Add half of the sliced peaches on top.

3. Repeat with the remaining cottage cheese and peaches.

4. Sprinkle with granola and drizzle with honey if desired.

5. Serve immediately and enjoy the delicious creamy and crunchy textures.

There is nothing quite like the comforting aroma of apples and cinnamon baking in the oven. This Baked Oatmeal with Apples and Cinnamon is a warm, hearty breakfast that feels like a cosy hug on a chilly morning. It's easy to make, nutritious, and perfect for a healthy start to your day.

Baked Oatmeal with Apples and Cinnamon

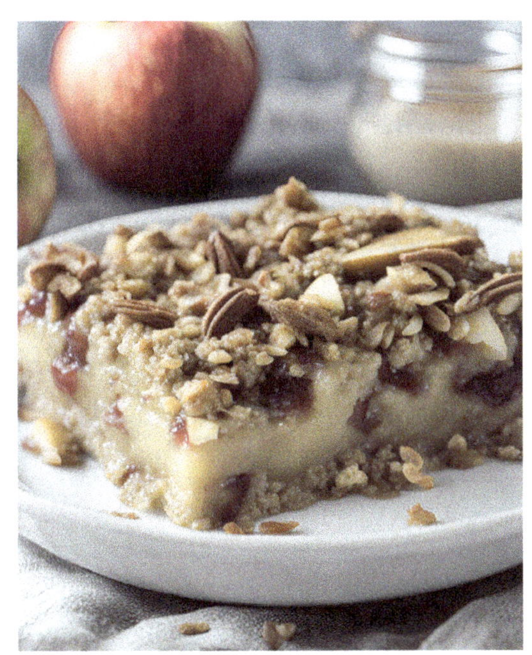

Preparation Time

Total: 45 minutes

Nutrition (per serving)

Calories: 180
Protein: 4g
Carbohydrates: 32g
Fiber: 5g
Fat: 4g

ingredients

- 2 cups rolled oats
- 1 1/2 cups unsweetened almond milk
- 2 apples, peeled and diced
- 1/4 cup unsweetened applesauce
- 1 teaspoon cinnamon
- 1 teaspoon vanilla extract
- 1/4 teaspoon salt
- Cooking spray

Instructions

1. Preheat your oven to 375°F (190°C).

2. Spray a baking dish with cooking spray.

3. combine the rolled oats, almond milk, apples, applesauce, cinnamon, vanilla extract, and salt in a large bowl.

4. Pour the mixture into the prepared baking dish and spread evenly.

5. Bake for 3540 minutes until the top is golden and the oatmeal is set.

6. Allow to cool slightly before serving. Enjoy it warm for a comforting breakfast treat.

Elevate your breakfast game with these elegant Poached Eggs over Asparagus Spears. This dish is not only visually stunning but also packed with nutrients. The tender asparagus pairs perfectly with the soft, runny poached eggs, making it a delightful and satisfying meal.

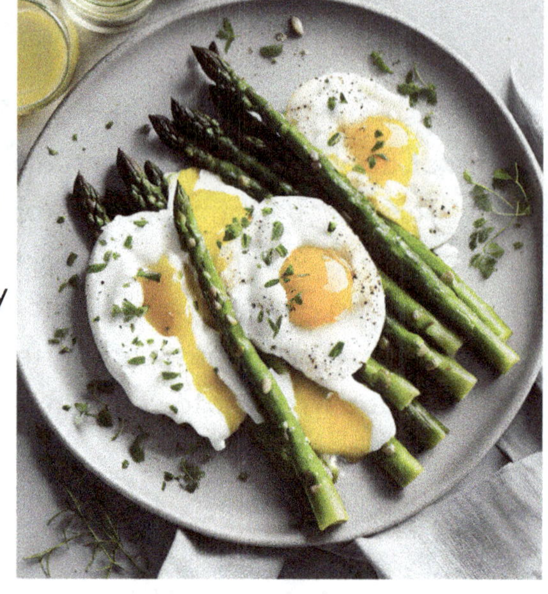

Poached Eggs over Asparagus Spears

Preparation Time

Total: 15 minutes

Nutrition (per serving)

Calories: 150
Protein: 12g
Carbohydrates: 5g
Fiber: 3g
Fat: 10g

ingredients

- 1 bunch of asparagus, trimmed
- 2 eggs
- 1 tablespoon white vinegar
- Salt and pepper to taste
- Cooking spray

Instructions

1. Fill a large skillet with water and bring to a simmer. Add the white vinegar.
2. Crack each egg into a small bowl.
3. Carefully slide the eggs into the simmering water and poach for 34 minutes until the whites are set but the yolks are still runny.
4. While the eggs are poaching, spray another skillet with cooking spray and heat over mediumhigh heat.
5. Add the asparagus and cook until tendercrisp, about 5 minutes.
6. Arrange the cooked asparagus on a plate and top with the poached eggs.
7. Season with salt and pepper and serve immediately.

About the recipe

This Sweet Potato and Black Bean Breakfast Burrito is a hearty and flavorful way to start your day. Packed with nutritious ingredients, it's a delicious, filling breakfast option for busy mornings or leisurely weekend brunch.

Sweet Potato and Black Bean Breakfast Burrito

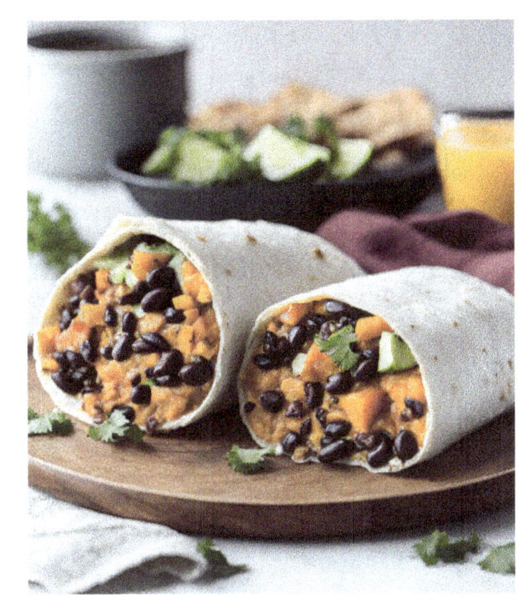

Preparation Time

Total: 25 minutes

Nutrition (per serving)

Calories: 250
Protein: 12g
Carbohydrates: 42g
Fiber: 8g
Fat: 6g

ingredients

- 1 medium sweet potato, peeled and diced
- 1/2 cup black beans, drained and rinsed
- 1 small onion, diced
- 1 bell pepper, diced
- 2 eggs
- 2 whole wheat tortillas
- Cooking spray
- Salt and pepper to taste

Instructions

1. Spray a skillet with cooking spray and heat over medium heat.
2. Add the sweet potato and cook until it softens, about 10 minutes.
3. Add the onion and bell pepper, cooking until all vegetables are tender, about five more minutes.
4. Stir in the black beans and cook until heated about 2 minutes.
5. In another skillet, scramble the eggs until just set, about 3 minutes.
6. Warm the tortillas in the microwave or skillet for 30 seconds.
7. Fill each tortilla with the sweet potato mixture and scrambled eggs, then roll into burritos. Serve immediately

34

About the recipe

These Zucchini and Carrot Muffins are a delightful way to sneak some veggies into your breakfast or snack. They are moist, flavorful, and nutritious, making them a perfect zeropoint treat

Zucchini and Carrot Muffins

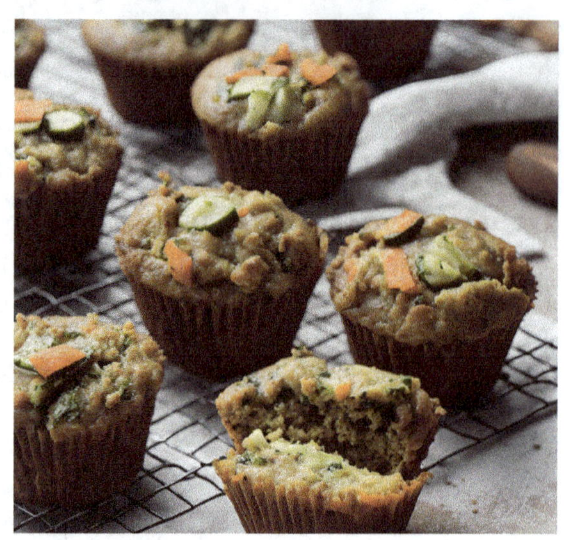

Preparation Time

Total: 35 minutes

Nutrition (per serving)

Calories: 100
Protein: 3g
Carbohydrates: 20g
Fiber: 3g
Fat: 2g

ingredients

- 1 cup grated zucchini
- 1 cup grated carrot
- 1 cup whole wheat flour
- 1/2 cup unsweetened applesauce
- 2 eggs
- 1 teaspoon baking powder
- 1/2 teaspoon baking soda
- 1 teaspoon cinnamon
- 1/2 teaspoon salt
- Cooking spray

Instructions

1. Preheat your oven to 350°F (175°C) and spray a muffin tin with cooking spray.
2. combine the grated zucchini, carrot, and applesauce in a large bowl.
3. Add the eggs and mix well.
4. whisk together the flour, baking powder, baking soda, cinnamon, and salt in a separate bowl.
5. Gradually add the dry ingredients to the wet ingredients, mixing until combined.
6. Divide the batter evenly among the muffin cups.
7. Bake for 2025 minutes or until a toothpick inserted into the centre comes clean.
8. Allow to cool before serving.

About the recipe

Start your day with a nutritious and satisfying Breakfast of Quinoa with Almond Milk. This warm and comforting bowl is packed with protein, fibre, and a hint of sweetness, making it the perfect way to fuel your morning

Breakfast Quinoa with Almond Milk

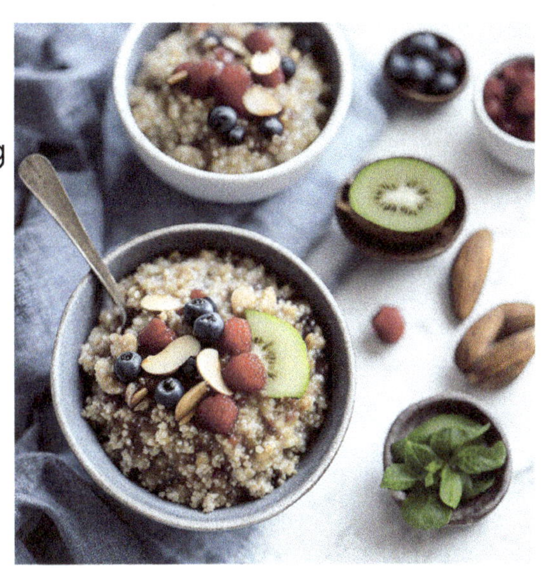

Preparation Time

Total: 20 minutes

Nutrition (per serving)

Calories: 220
Protein: 6g
Carbohydrates: 36g
Fiber: 6g
Fat: 6g

ingredients

- 1/2 cup quinoa, rinsed
- 1 cup unsweetened almond milk
- 1 tablespoon chia seeds
- 1 tablespoon honey (optional)
- 1/2 teaspoon vanilla extract
- Fresh fruit for topping (such as berries, banana slices, or apple chunks)

Instructions

1. In a medium saucepan, combine the quinoa and almond milk. Bring to a boil.

2. Reduce the heat to low, cover, and simmer for 15 minutes until the quinoa is tender and the liquid is absorbed.

3. Stir in the chia seeds, honey (if using), and vanilla extract.

4. Spoon the quinoa into bowls and top with fresh fruit.

5. Serve warm and enjoy a hearty, healthy breakfast.

CHAPTER THREE

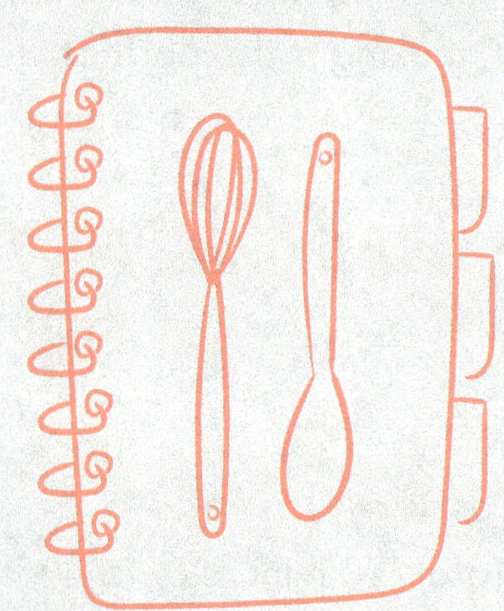

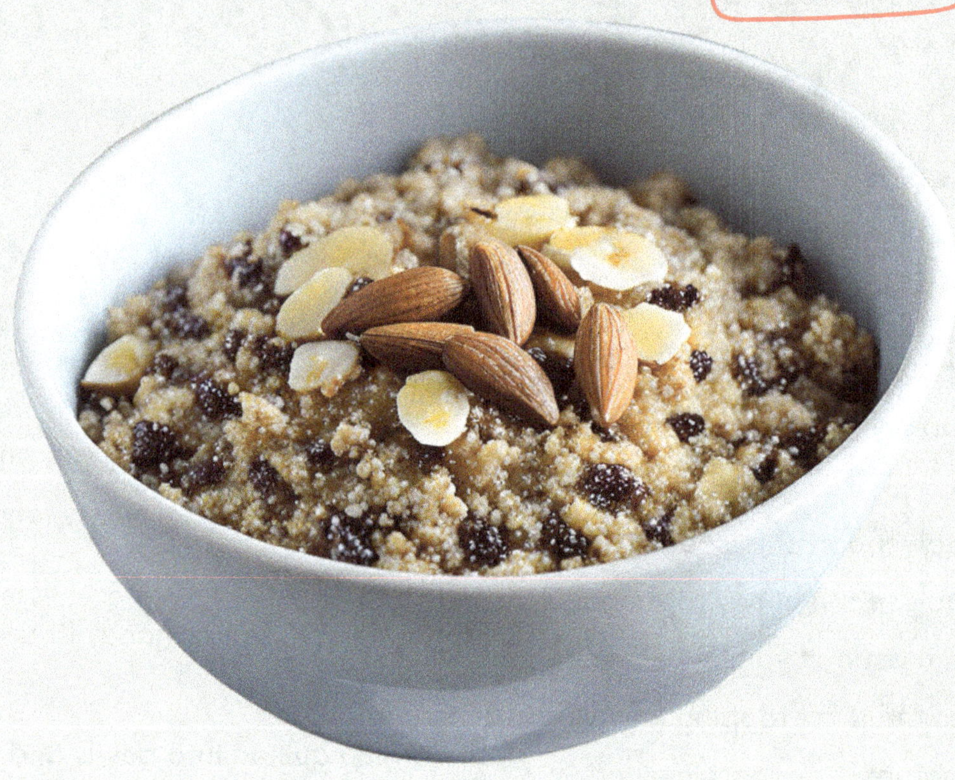

lunch Recipes

Craving something crispy and delicious but want to keep it healthy? These Sweet Potato Fries with Avocado Dip are the perfect solution! Baked to perfection, these fries are a guiltfree treat, and the creamy avocado dip adds a refreshing twist.

Sweet Potato Fries with Avocado Dip

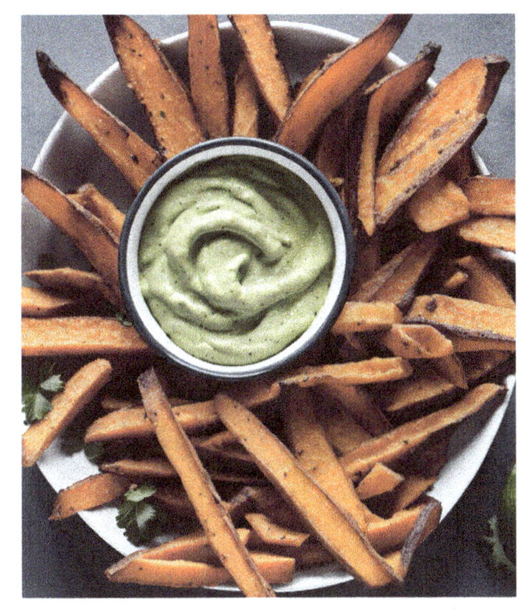

Preparation Time

Total: 35 minutes

Nutrition (per serving)

Calories: 180
Protein: 3g
Carbohydrates: 30g
Fiber: 6g
Fat: 7g

ingredients

For the Fries:

- 2 large sweet potatoes, peeled and cut into thin fries
- 1 tablespoon olive oil
- 1 teaspoon paprika
- 1/2 teaspoon garlic powder
- Salt and pepper to taste

For the Avocado Dip:

- 1 ripe avocado
- 1/4 cup Greek yogurt
- 1 tablespoon lime juice
- Salt and pepper to taste

Instructions

1. Preheat your oven to 425°F (220°C).

2. In a large bowl, toss the sweet potato fries with olive oil, paprika, garlic powder, salt, and pepper.

3. Spread the fries in a single layer on a baking sheet lined with parchment paper.

4. Bake for 2530 minutes, turning halfway through, until crispy and golden.

5. While the fries are baking, prepare the avocado dip. In a small bowl, mash the avocado and mix with Greek yoghurt, lime juice, salt, and pepper until smooth.

6. Serve the sweet potato fries with the avocado dip on the side.

About the recipe

This Greek Salad with Lemon Dressing is a vibrant and refreshing starter that is perfect for any meal. Packed with crunchy vegetables and a zesty lemon dressing, it's a burst of flavours that will tantalize your taste buds.

Greek Salad with Lemon Dressing

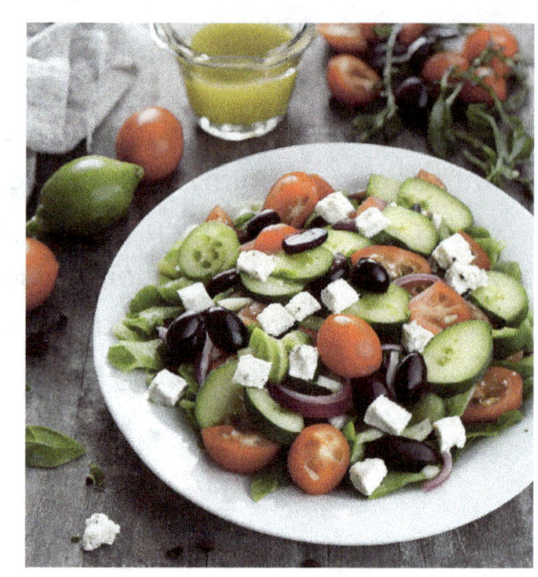

Preparation Time

Total: 15 minutes

Nutrition (per serving)

Calories: 120
Protein: 2g
Carbohydrates: 8g
Fiber: 3g
Fat: 10g

ingredients

For the Salad:

2 cups chopped romaine lettuce
1 cucumber, diced
1 bell pepper, diced
1/2 red onion, thinly sliced
1/2 cup cherry tomatoes, halved
1/4 cup Kalamata olives
1/4 cup crumbled feta cheese (optional)

For the Lemon Dressing:

1/4 cup olive oil
2 tablespoons lemon juice
1 teaspoon dried oregano
Salt and pepper to taste

Instructions

1. Combine the romaine lettuce, cucumber, bell pepper, red onion, cherry tomatoes, and Kalamata olives in a large salad bowl.

2. To make the dressing, whisk together the olive oil, lemon juice, dried oregano, salt, and pepper in a small bowl.

3. Pour the dressing over the salad and toss to combine.

4. Sprinkle with crumbled feta cheese, if desired, and serve immediately.

About the recipe

This Spinach and Artichoke Dip is a delicious appetizer to share. Made with wholesome ingredients, it's a healthier take on a classic favourite. Serve it with wholegrain crackers or fresh veggies for dipping.

Spinach and Artichoke Dip

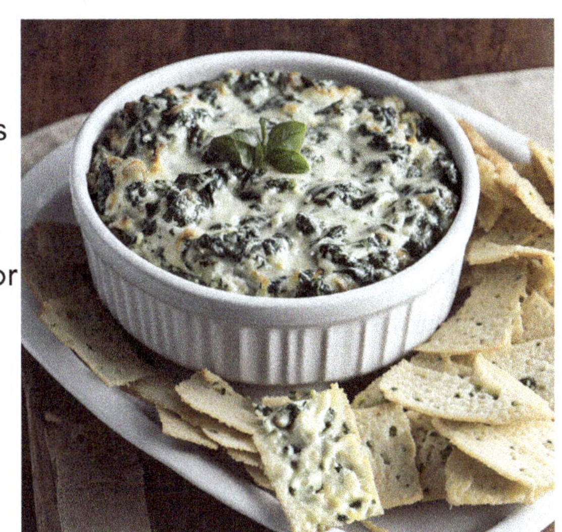

Preparation Time

Total: 30 minutes

Nutrition (per serving)

Calories: 150
Protein: 10g
Carbohydrates: 5g
Fiber: 2g
Fat: 10g

ingredients

- 1 cup Greek yogurt
- 1/2 cup grated Parmesan cheese
- 1/2 cup mozzarella cheese, shredded
- 1 cup canned artichoke hearts, drained and chopped
- 1 cup fresh spinach, chopped
- 2 cloves garlic, minced
- Salt and pepper to taste

Instructions

1. Preheat your oven to 375°F (190°C).

2. Mix the Greek yoghurt, Parmesan cheese, mozzarella cheese, artichoke hearts, spinach, garlic, salt, and pepper in a mixing bowl.

3. Transfer the mixture to a baking dish.

4. Bake for 2025 minutes until the dip is bubbly and golden on top.

5. Serve warm with wholegrain crackers or fresh veggies.

About the recipe

Are you looking for a crunchy snack that's also good for you? These Baked Kale Chips are the answer! They're crispy, flavorful, and straightforward to make, perfect for a quick snack or as a healthy appetizer.

Baked Kale Chips

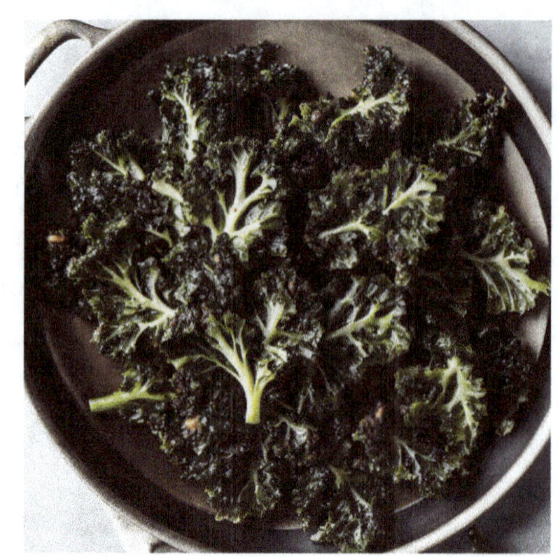

Preparation Time
Total: 20 minutes

Nutrition (per serving)
Calories: 50
Protein: 2g
Carbohydrates: 7g
Fiber: 3g
Fat: 2g

ingredients

- 1 bunch of kale, washed and dried
- 1 tablespoon olive oil
- 1/2 teaspoon salt
- 1/4 teaspoon garlic powder (optional)

Instructions

1. Preheat your oven to 350°F (175°C).

2. Remove the kale leaves from the stems and tear them into bitesized pieces.

3. In a large bowl, toss the kale with olive oil, salt, and garlic powder (if using).

4. Spread the kale leaves in a single layer on a baking sheet lined with parchment paper.

5. Bake for 1015 minutes until the edges are browned and crispy.

6. Let cool slightly before serving.

About the recipe

These Spicy Roasted Chickpeas are a crunchy and flavorful snack perfect for munching. They're easy to make, packed with protein, and can be seasoned to suit your taste. Enjoy them as a snack or a fun appetizer.

Spicy Roasted Chickpeas

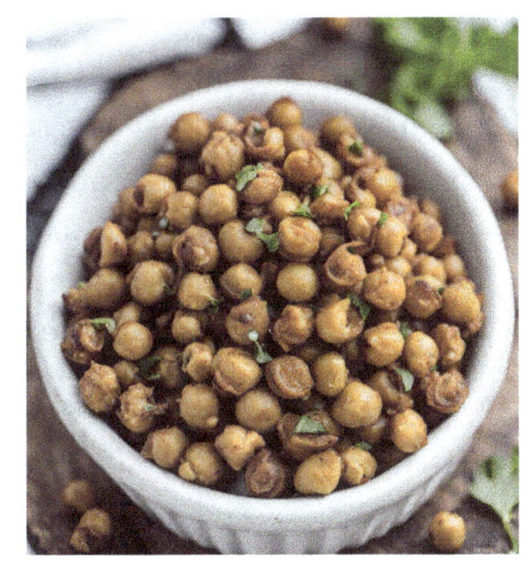

Preparation Time

Total: 30 minutes

Nutrition (per serving)

Calories: 120
Protein: 5g
Carbohydrates: 18g
Fiber: 6g
Fat: 4g

ingredients

- 1 can chickpeas, drained and rinsed
- 1 tablespoon olive oil
- 1 teaspoon paprika
- 1/2 teaspoon cumin
- 1/4 teaspoon cayenne pepper
- 1/2 teaspoon salt

Instructions

1. Preheat your oven to 400°F (200°C).

2. Pat the chickpeas dry with a paper towel.

3. toss the chickpeas with olive oil, paprika, cumin, cayenne pepper, and salt in a bowl.

4. Spread the chickpeas in a single layer on a baking sheet lined with parchment paper.

5. Roast for 2025 minutes, shaking the pan halfway through, until the chickpeas are crispy and golden.

6. Let cool before serving.

About the recipe

Zucchini Noodles with Pesto is a light and refreshing starter that's both delicious and nutritious. Spiralized zucchini replaces traditional pasta, making this dish low in carbs but high in flavour. The fresh pesto adds a delightful, aromatic touch.

Zucchini Noodles with Pesto

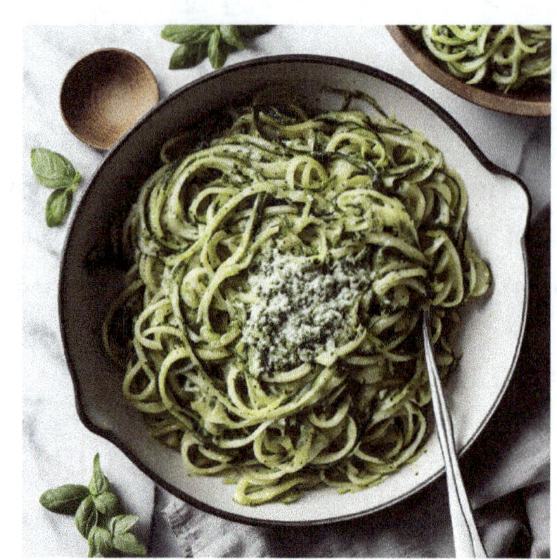

Preparation Time

Total: 15 minutes

Nutrition (per serving)

Calories: 180
Protein: 5g
Carbohydrates: 8g
Fiber: 2g
Fat: 16g

ingredients

- 2 medium zucchinis, spiralized
- 1 cup fresh basil leaves
- 1/4 cup pine nuts
- 1/4 cup grated Parmesan cheese
- 1 garlic clove
- 1/4 cup olive oil
- Salt and pepper to taste

Instructions

1. combine the basil, pine nuts, Parmesan cheese, and garlic in a food processor. Pulse until finely chopped.

2. Slowly add the olive oil until the mixture is smooth and the processor is running. Season with salt and pepper.

3. In a large bowl, toss the spiralized zucchini with the pesto until evenly coated.

4. Serve immediately as a fresh and vibrant starter.

About the recipe

These Stuffed Mini Bell Peppers are colourful, bitesized treats perfect for any occasion. Filled with a creamy, herby mixture, they are delicious but also healthy and satisfying. It's ideal as a starter or a light snack!

Stuffed Mini Bell Peppers

Preparation Time

Total: 30 minutes

Nutrition (per serving)

Nutrition (per serving):
Calories: 50
Protein: 2g
Carbohydrates: 4g
Fiber: 1g
Fat: 3g

ingredients

- 12 mini bell peppers
- 1 cup lowfat cream cheese
- 1/4 cup finely chopped fresh herbs (parsley, chives, and dill)
- 1 garlic clove, minced
- Salt and pepper to taste

Instructions

1. Preheat your oven to 375°F (190°C).

2. Slice the tops of the mini bell peppers and remove the seeds.

3. mix the lowfat cream cheese, chopped herbs, minced garlic, salt, and pepper until well combined.

4. Spoon the mixture into the mini bell peppers.

5. Place the stuffed peppers on a baking sheet lined with parchment paper.

6. Bake for 1520 minutes, until the peppers are tender and the filling is slightly golden.

7. Serve warm or at room temperature.

About the recipe

This Watermelon and Feta Salad is a refreshing and delightful starter that combines sweet, juicy watermelon with salty feta cheese and a hint of mint. It's a perfect summer dish that's light, flavorful, and incredibly easy to make.

Watermelon and Feta Salad

Preparation Time

Total: 10 minutes

Nutrition (per serving)

Calories: 120
Protein: 4g
Carbohydrates: 12g
Fiber: 1g
Fat: 8g

ingredients

- 4 cups cubed watermelon
- 1/2 cup crumbled feta cheese
- 1/4 cup fresh mint leaves, chopped
- 2 tablespoons olive oil
- 1 tablespoon balsamic vinegar
- Salt and pepper to taste

Instructions

1. combine the cubed watermelon, crumbled feta, and chopped mint leaves in a large bowl.

2. Drizzle with olive oil and balsamic vinegar.

3. Gently toss to combine.

4. Season with salt and pepper to taste.

5. Serve immediately for a relaxed and refreshing starter.

About the recipe

These Caprese Skewers with Balsamic Glaze are a fun and elegant way to serve a classic Italian favourite. Featuring fresh mozzarella, cherry tomatoes, and basil leaves, these skewers are drizzled with a tangy balsamic glaze, making them a hit at any gathering.

Caprese Skewers with Balsamic Glaze

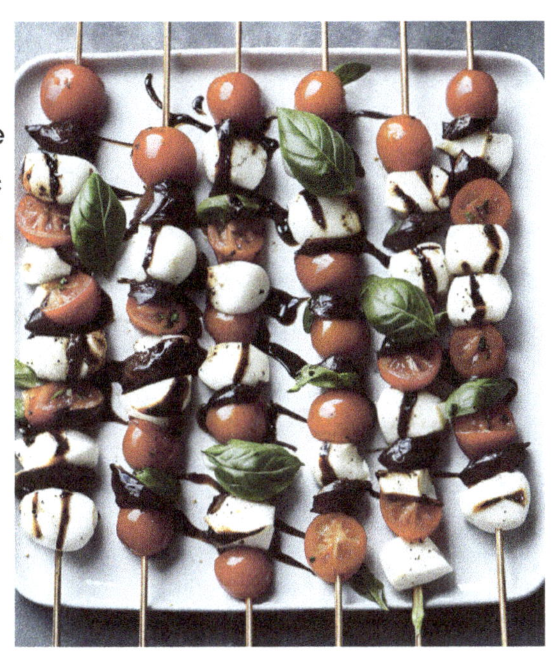

Preparation Time

Total: 15 minutes

Nutrition (per serving)

Calories: 90
Protein: 5g
Carbohydrates: 6g
Fiber: 1g
Fat: 5g

ingredients

- 20 cherry tomatoes
- 20 small fresh mozzarella balls
- 20 fresh basil leaves
- 1/4 cup balsamic vinegar
- 1 tablespoon honey
- 20 small skewers

Instructions

1. Combine the balsamic vinegar and honey in a small saucepan. Bring to a simmer over medium heat and cook until reduced by half and slightly thickened, about 57 minutes. Set aside to cool.

2. Thread one cherry tomato, mozzarella ball, and basil leaf onto each skewer.

3. Arrange the skewers on a serving platter.

4. Drizzle the balsamic glaze over the skewers just before serving.

About the recipe

Roasted Brussels Sprouts with Garlic is a simple yet delicious starter or side dish. The Brussels sprouts become crispy and caramelized in the oven, and the garlic adds a beautiful depth of flavour.

Roasted Brussels sprouts with Garlic

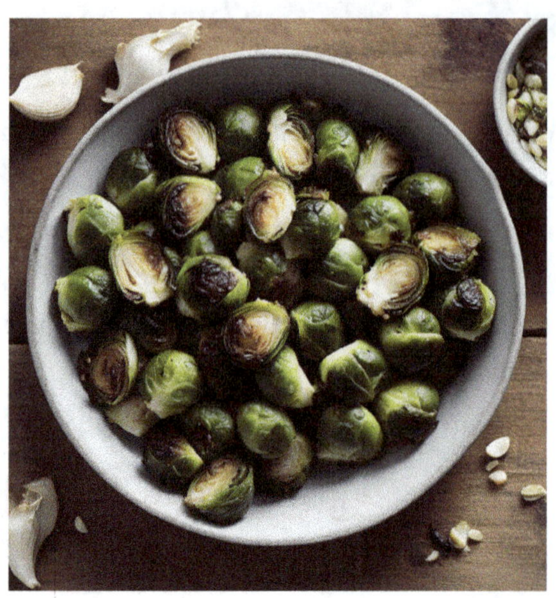

Preparation Time

Total: 30 minutes

Nutrition (per serving)

Calories: 110
Protein: 3g
Carbohydrates: 10g
Fiber: 4g
Fat: 7g

ingredients

- 1 lb Brussels sprouts, trimmed and halved
- 2 tablespoons olive oil
- 3 garlic cloves, minced
- Salt and pepper to taste

Instructions

1. Preheat your oven to 400°F (200°C).

2. toss the Brussels sprouts with olive oil, minced garlic, salt, and pepper in a large bowl.

3. Spread the Brussels sprouts in a single layer on a baking sheet lined with parchment paper.

4. Roast for 2025 minutes, stirring halfway through, until golden brown and crispy.

5. Serve hot and enjoy the delicious flavors.

About the recipe

This Tomato Basil Soup is a comforting and flavorful starter for any time of the year. Made with fresh tomatoes and fragrant basil, it's light, healthy, and vibrant.

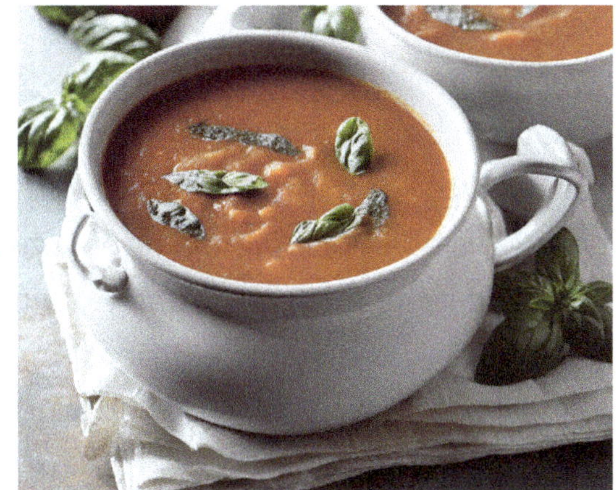

Tomato Basil Soup

Preparation Time

Total: 35 minutes

Nutrition (per serving)

Calories: 120
Protein: 2g
Carbohydrates: 15g
Fiber: 3g
Fat: 7g

ingredients

- 2 tablespoons olive oil
- 1 onion, chopped
- 3 garlic cloves, minced
- 6 large tomatoes, chopped
- 2 cups vegetable broth
- 1/4 cup fresh basil leaves, chopped
- Salt and pepper to taste

Instructions

1. heat the olive oil over medium heat in a large pot.
2. Add the chopped onion and cook until softened about 5 minutes.
3. Add the garlic and cook for another minute.
4. Add the chopped tomatoes and cook until they break down, about 10 minutes.
5. Pour in the vegetable broth and bring to a simmer.
6. Cook for 1520 minutes until the flavours have melded.
7. Use an immersion blender to blend the soup until smooth.
8. Stir in the chopped basil and season with salt and pepper.
9. Serve hot and enjoy the fresh flavours of this comforting soup.

About the recipe

Cucumber and Mint Gazpacho is a refreshing, light starter perfect for warm days. This chilled soup is made with fresh cucumbers, mint, and a hint of lime, offering a burst of extraordinary hydrating and delicious flavours.

Cucumber and Mint Gazpacho

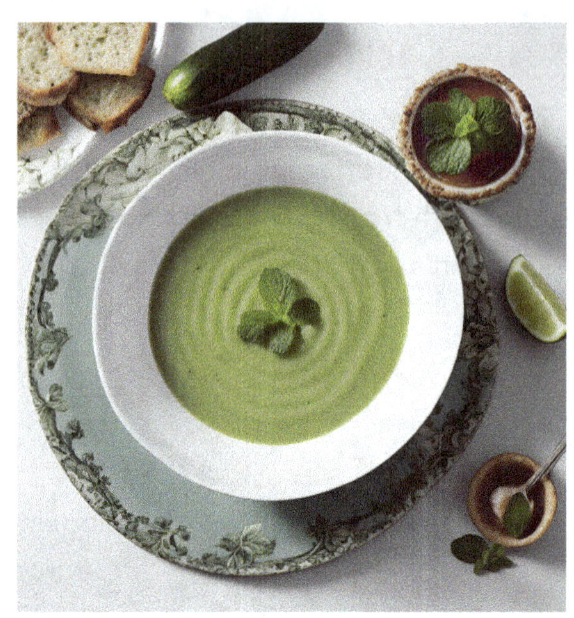

Preparation Time

Total: 15 minutes
(plus 1 hour chilling time)

Nutrition (per serving)

Calories: 70
Protein: 3g
Carbohydrates: 10g
Fiber: 2g
Fat: 2g

ingredients

- 2 large cucumbers, peeled and chopped
- 1/2 cup Greek yogurt
- 1/4 cup fresh mint leaves
- 2 tablespoons lime juice
- 1 garlic clove, minced
- Salt and pepper to taste

Instructions

1. combine the chopped cucumbers, Greek yoghurt, mint leaves, lime juice, and minced garlic in a blender.

2. Blend until smooth.

3. Season with salt and pepper to taste.

4. Chill in the refrigerator for at least 1 hour before serving.

5. Serve cold, garnished with extra mint leaves if desired.

About the recipe

This Grilled Peach and Mozzarella Salad is a delightful combination of sweet, juicy peaches and creamy mozzarella, all brought together with a fresh, tangy dressing. Perfect for summer, this salad is light, refreshing, and incredibly satisfying.

Grilled Peach and Mozzarella Salad

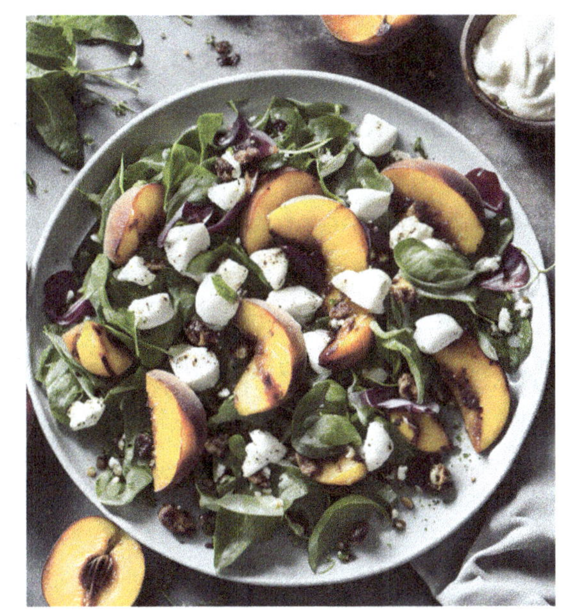

Preparation Time

Total: 15 minutes

Nutrition (per serving)

Calories: 150
Protein: 8g
Carbohydrates: 12g
Fiber: 3g
Fat: 9g

ingredients

- 2 ripe peaches, halved and pitted
- 4 oz fresh mozzarella, sliced
- 4 cups mixed greens
- 1/4 cup fresh basil leaves
- 2 tablespoons balsamic glaze
- 1 tablespoon olive oil
- Salt and pepper to taste

Instructions

1. Preheat your grill to mediumhigh heat.
2. Brush the peach halves with olive oil and place them on the grill, cutting the side down. Grill for 34 minutes until they have excellent grill marks and are slightly softened.
3. Remove the peaches from the grill and let them cool slightly before slicing.
4. combine the mixed greens, grilled peach slices, mozzarella, and basil leaves in a large salad bowl.
5. Drizzle with balsamic glaze, sprinkle with salt and pepper, and toss gently to combine.
6. Serve immediately and enjoy the perfect balance of sweet and savoury flavours.

About the recipe

Bright and refreshing, this Avocado and Grapefruit Salad is a perfect starter for any meal. The creamy avocado pairs beautifully with the tartness of the grapefruit, creating a delicious and nutritious dish that's visually appealing and tasty.

Avocado and Grapefruit Salad

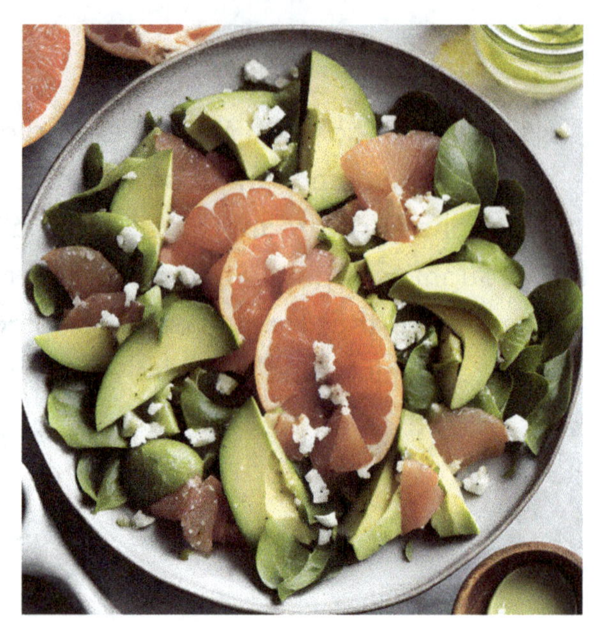

Preparation Time

Total: 10 minutes

Nutrition (per serving) 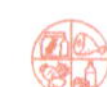

Calories: 180
Protein: 2g
Carbohydrates: 15g
Fiber: 8g
Fat: 14g

ingredients

- 2 ripe avocados, peeled, pitted, and sliced
- 2 grapefruits, peeled and segmented
- 4 cups mixed greens
- 1/4 cup red onion, thinly sliced
- 2 tablespoons olive oil
- 1 tablespoon lime juice
- Salt and pepper to taste

Instructions

1. Combine the mixed greens, avocado slices, grapefruit segments, and red onion in a large salad bowl.

2. Whisk together the olive oil, lime juice, salt, and pepper in a small bowl.

3. Drizzle the dressing over the salad and toss gently to combine.

4. Serve immediately for a refreshing and light starter.

About the recipe

This Carrot and Coriander Soup is a warm, comforting starter that's both healthy and delicious. The sweet carrots and aromatic coriander create a perfect blend of flavours, making this soup a delightful way to start any meal.

Carrot and Coriander Soup

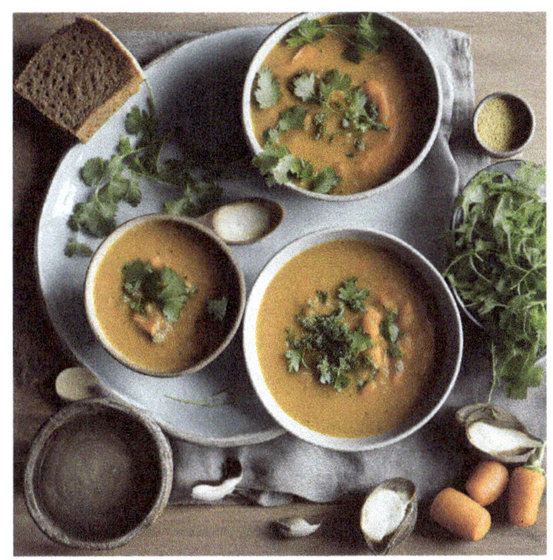

Preparation Time

Total: 30 minutes

Nutrition (per serving)

Calories: 120
Protein: 2g
Carbohydrates: 18g
Fiber: 5g
Fat: 4g

ingredients

- 1 tablespoon olive oil
- 1 onion, chopped
- 2 garlic cloves, minced
- 6 large carrots, peeled and chopped
- 4 cups vegetable broth
- 1 teaspoon ground coriander
- 1/4 cup fresh coriander leaves, chopped
- Salt and pepper to taste

Instructions

1. Heat the olive oil over medium heat in a large pot.
2. Add the chopped onion and cook until softened about 5 minutes.
3. Add the minced garlic and cook for another minute.
4. Stir in the chopped carrots and ground coriander, cooking for a few more minutes.
5. Pour in the vegetable broth and bring to a boil.
6. Reduce the heat and simmer for 20 minutes until the carrots are tender.
7. Use an immersion blender to blend the soup until smooth.
8. Stir in the fresh coriander leaves and season with salt and pepper.
9. Serve hot, garnished with extra coriander leaves if desired.

About the recipe

This Beetroot and Goat Cheese Salad is a colourful and flavorful starter that's sure to impress. The earthy sweetness of the beetroot combined with the creamy tang of goat cheese makes for a delightful and nutritious dish.

Beetroot and Goat Cheese Salad

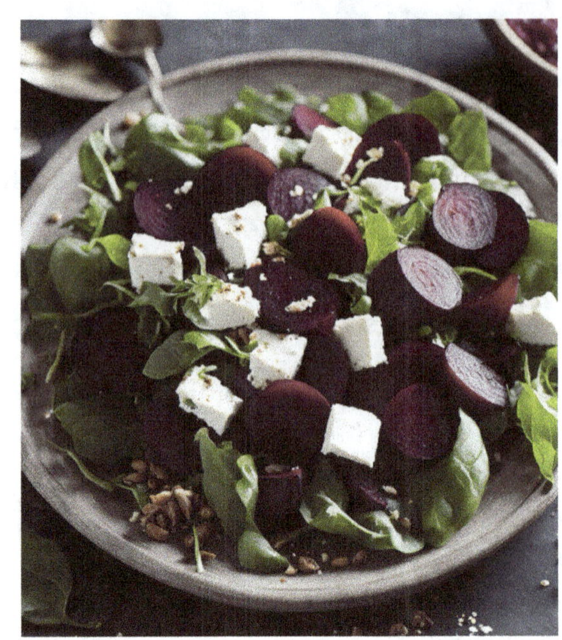

Preparation Time

Total: 60 minutes
(including roasting time)

Nutrition (per serving)

Calories: 200
Protein: 6g
Carbohydrates: 15g
Fiber: 5g
Fat: 14g

ingredients

- 4 medium beets, roasted and sliced
- 4 oz goat cheese, crumbled
- 4 cups mixed greens
- 1/4 cup walnuts, toasted and chopped
- 2 tablespoons balsamic vinegar
- 1 tablespoon olive oil
- Salt and pepper to taste

Instructions

1. Preheat your oven to 400°F (200°C). Wrap each beet in foil and roast for 4560 minutes until tender. Let cool before peeling and slicing.
2. Combine the mixed greens, roasted beet slices, crumbled goat cheese, and toasted walnuts in a large salad bowl.
3. Whisk together the balsamic vinegar, olive oil, salt, and pepper in a small bowl.
4. Drizzle the dressing over the salad and toss gently to combine.
5. Serve immediately and enjoy the beautiful medley of flavors.

About the recipe

Edamame with Sea Salt is a simple, healthy, and delicious starter that is perfect for any occasion. These young soybeans are packed with protein and fibre, making them a satisfying and nutritious snack.

Edamame with Sea Salt

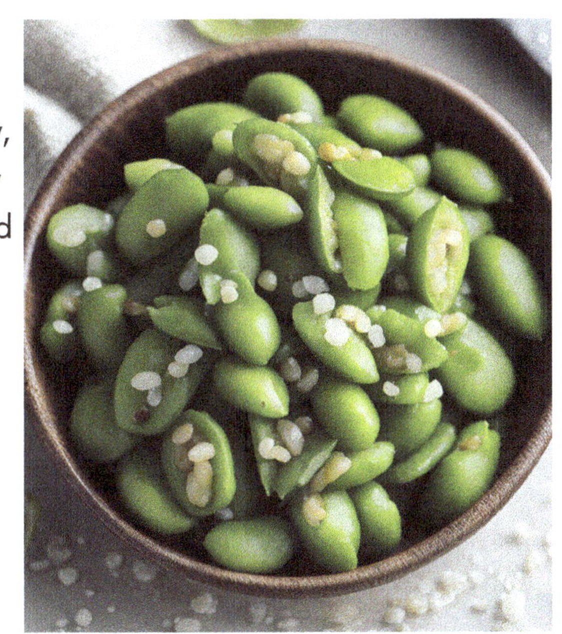

Preparation Time

Total: 10 minutes

Nutrition (per serving)

Calories: 100
Protein: 8g
Carbohydrates: 8g
Fiber: 4g
Fat: 4g

ingredients

- 2 cups edamame in the pod
- 1 tablespoon sea salt

Instructions

1. Bring a large pot of water to a boil.

2. Add the edamame and cook for 5 minutes until tender.

3. Drain the edamame and transfer to a serving bowl.

4. Sprinkle with sea salt and toss to coat.

5. Serve immediately and enjoy!

About the recipe

Cauliflower Buffalo Bites are a spicy and healthy alternative to traditional buffalo wings. These crispy, flavorful bites are perfect for a gameday snack or a fun appetizer, and they're sure to be a hit with everyone.

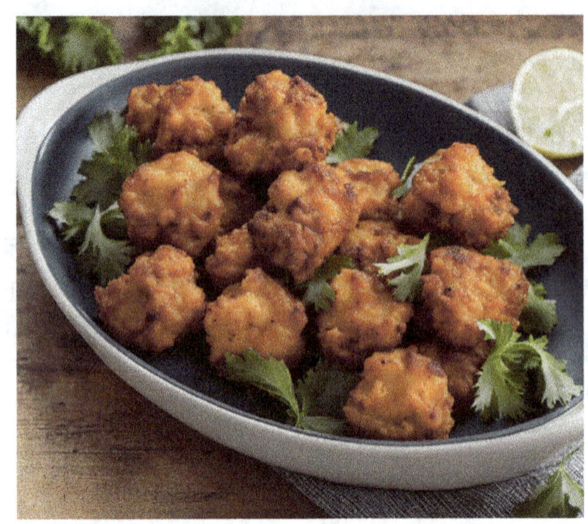

Cauliflower Buffalo Bites

Preparation Time

Total: 35 minutes

Nutrition (per serving)

Calories: 90
Protein: 3g
Carbohydrates: 12g
Fiber: 4g
Fat: 4g

ingredients

- 1 head cauliflower, cut into bitesized florets
- 1/2 cup whole wheat flour
- 1/2 cup water
- 1/2 teaspoon garlic powder
- 1/2 teaspoon paprika
- 1/4 teaspoon salt
- 1/4 cup hot sauce
- 1 tablespoon olive oil

Instructions

1. Preheat your oven to 450°F (230°C) and line a baking sheet with parchment paper.
2. whisk the flour, water, garlic powder, paprika, and salt in a large bowl until smooth.
3. Add the cauliflower florets to the bowl and toss to coat evenly.
4. Spread the coated cauliflower on the prepared baking sheet and bake for 20 minutes.
5. mix the hot Sauce and olive oil in a small bowl.
6. Remove the cauliflower from the oven and brush with the hot sauce mixture.
7. Return to the oven and bake for 10 minutes until crispy.
8. Serve immediately with your favourite dipping sauce.

About the recipe

Warm up with this creamy, nutritious Broccoli and Almond Soup. Packed with vitamins and a delightful nutty flavour, this soup is delicious and a zeropoint treat that will keep you full and satisfied.

Broccoli and Almond Soup

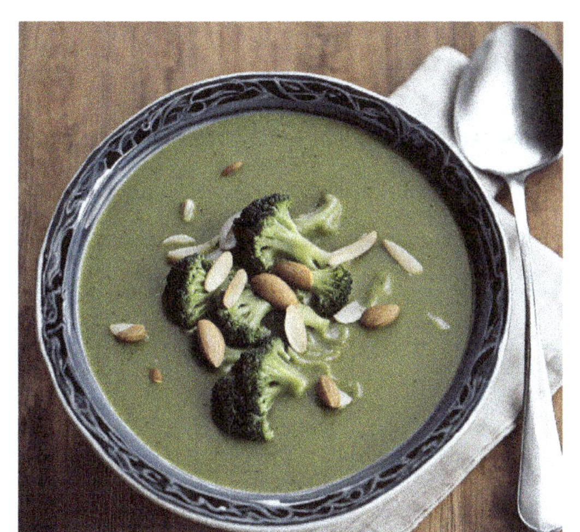

Preparation Time

Total: 30 minutes

Nutrition (per serving)

Calories: 120
Protein: 4g
Carbohydrates: 12g
Fiber: 4g
Fat: 7g

ingredients

- 1 tablespoon olive oil
- 1 onion, chopped
- 2 garlic cloves, minced
- 4 cups broccoli florets
- 1/4 cup sliced almonds
- 4 cups vegetable broth
- Salt and pepper to taste
- 1/4 cup almond milk (optional)

Instructions

1. heat the olive oil over medium heat in a large pot.
2. Add the chopped onion and cook until softened about 5 minutes.
3. Add the minced garlic and cook for another minute.
4. Stir in the broccoli florets and sliced almonds, cooking for a few more minutes.
5. Pour in the vegetable broth and bring to a boil.
6. Reduce the heat and simmer for 1520 minutes until the broccoli is tender.
7. Use an immersion blender to blend the soup until smooth. Stir in the almond milk if using.
8. Season with salt and pepper to taste.
9. Serve hot, garnished with extra sliced almonds if desired.

About the recipe

This Arugula and Parmesan Salad is a simple yet elegant starter bursting with flavour. The peppery arugula paired with the sharpness of Parmesan and a zesty lemon dressing makes for a refreshing and delightful dish.

Arugula and Parmesan Salad

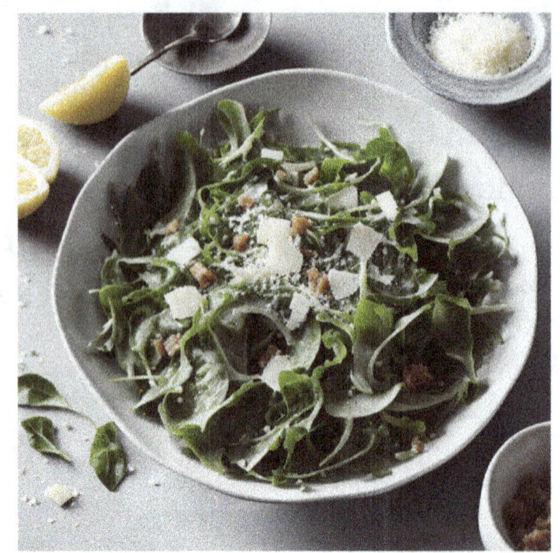

Preparation Time

Total: 5 minutes

Nutrition (per serving)

Calories: 80
Protein: 4g
Carbohydrates: 2g
Fiber: 1g
Fat: 7g

ingredients

- 4 cups fresh arugula
- 1/4 cup shaved Parmesan cheese
- 1 tablespoon olive oil
- 1 tablespoon lemon juice
- Salt and pepper to taste

Instructions

1. Combine the fresh arugula and shaved Parmesan cheese in a large salad bowl.
2. Whisk together the olive oil, lemon juice, salt, and pepper in a small bowl.
3. Drizzle the dressing over the salad and toss gently to combine.
4. Serve immediately for a crisp and flavorful start to your meal.

About the recipe

If you're looking for a light, refreshing, and incredibly nutritious salad, looks no further! This Lemon Herb Quinoa Salad is a perfect blend of tangy lemon, fresh herbs, and wholesome quinoa.

Lemon Herb Quinoa Salad

Preparation Time

Total:30 minutes

Nutrition (per serving)

Calories 180
Protein 6g
Carbohydrates 28g
Fiber 5g
Fat 6g
Sodium: 20mg

ingredients

- 1 cup quinoa, rinsed
- 2 cups water or vegetable broth
- 1 cup cherry tomatoes, halved
- 1 cucumber, diced
- 1 red bell pepper, diced
- 1/4 cup red onion, finely chopped
- 1/4 cup fresh parsley, chopped
- 1/4 cup fresh mint, chopped
- 1/4 cup fresh basil, chopped
- Juice of 2 lemons
- 2 tablespoons extra virgin olive oil
- Salt and pepper to taste

Instructions

1, In a medium saucepan, bring the quinoa and water or vegetable broth to a boil. Reduce the heat to low, cover,

2. While the quinoa is cooling, prepare the cherry tomatoes, cucumber, red bell pepper, and red onion. Combine them in a large mixing bowl.

3. Finely chop the parsley, mint, and basil. Add them to the bowl with the vegetables.

4. In a small bowl, whisk together the lemon juice, olive oil, salt, and pepper.

5. Add the cooled quinoa to the bowl with the vegetables and herbs. Pour the dressing over the salad and toss well to combine. Adjust the seasoning with more salt and pepper if needed.

About the recipe

This Greek Salad with Lemon Dressing is a vibrant and refreshing starter that is perfect for any meal. Packed with crunchy vegetables and a zesty lemon dressing, it's a burst of flavours that will tantalize your taste buds.

Greek Salad with Lemon Dressing

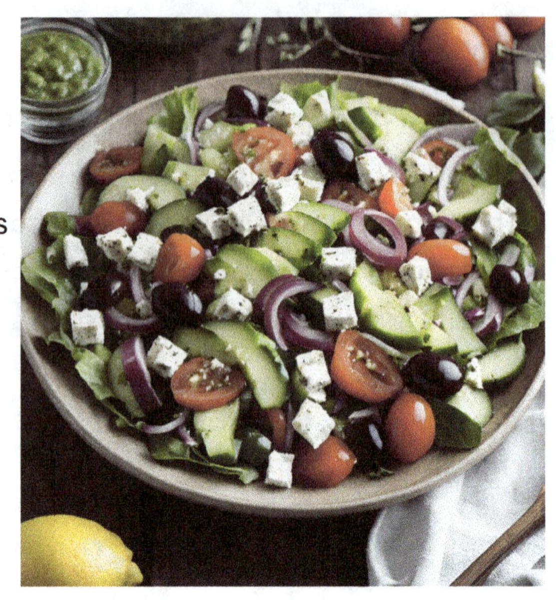

Preparation Time

Total: 15 minutes

Nutrition (per serving)

Calories: 120
Protein: 2g
Carbohydrates: 8g
Fiber: 3g
Fat: 10g

ingredients

For the Salad:

- 2 cups chopped romaine lettuce
- 1 cucumber, diced
- 1 bell pepper, diced
- 1/2 red onion, thinly sliced
- 1/2 cup cherry tomatoes, halved
- 1/4 cup Kalamata olives
- 1/4 cup crumbled feta cheese (optional)

For the Lemon Dressing:

- 1/4 cup olive oil
- 2 tablespoons lemon juice
- 1 teaspoon dried oregano
- Salt and pepper to taste

Instructions

1. combine the romaine lettuce, cucumber, bell pepper, red onion, cherry tomatoes, and Kalamata olives in a large salad bowl.
2. To make the dressing, whisk together the olive oil, lemon juice, dried oregano, salt, and pepper in a small bowl.
3. Pour the dressing over the salad and toss to combine.
4. Sprinkle with crumbled feta cheese, if desired, and serve immediately.

This Spinach and Artichoke Dip is a delicious appetizer to share. Made with wholesome ingredients, it's a healthier take on a classic favourite. Serve it with wholegrain crackers or fresh veggies for dipping.

Spinach and Artichoke Dip

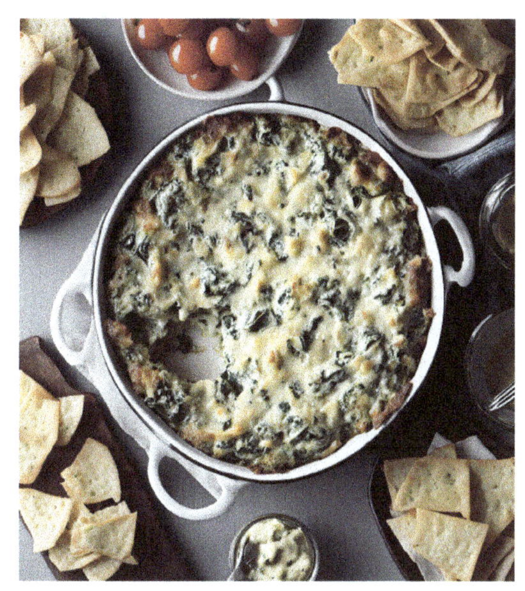

Preparation Time

Total: 30 minutes

Nutrition (per serving)

Calories: 150
Protein: 10g
Carbohydrates: 5g
Fiber: 2g
Fat: 10g

ingredients

1 cup Greek yogurt
1/2 cup grated Parmesan cheese
1/2 cup mozzarella cheese, shredded
1 cup canned artichoke hearts, drained and chopped
1 cup fresh spinach, chopped
2 cloves garlic, minced
Salt and pepper to taste

Instructions

1. Preheat your oven to 375°F (190°C).
2. Mix the Greek yoghurt, Parmesan cheese, mozzarella cheese, artichoke hearts, spinach, garlic, salt, and pepper in a mixing bowl.
3. Transfer the mixture to a baking dish.
4. Bake for 2025 minutes until the dip is bubbly and golden on top.
5. Serve warm with wholegrain crackers or fresh veggies.

CHAPTER FOUR

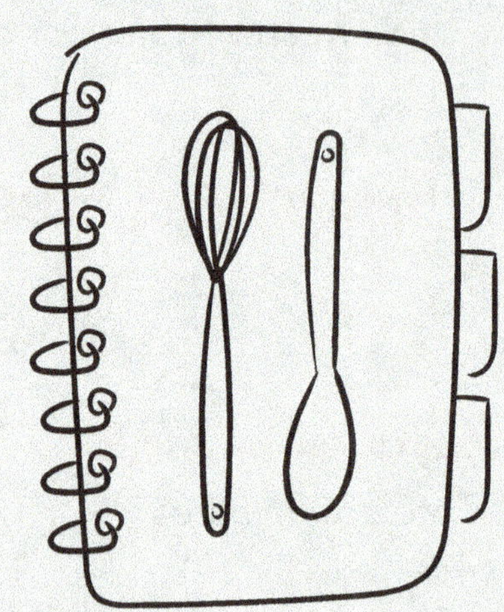

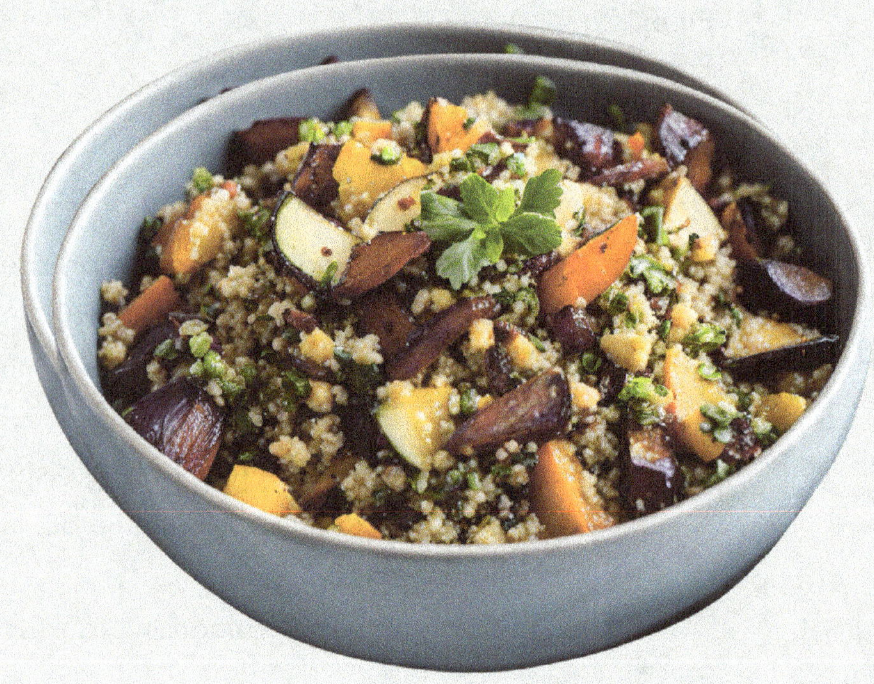

Dinner recipes

Enjoy a delightful, protein packed meal with this Grilled Chicken with Quinoa and Avocado Salad. The juicy grilled chicken pairs perfectly with the nutty quinoa and creamy avocado, making for a satisfying and nutritious dish bursting with fresh flavors.

Grilled Chicken with Quinoa and Avocado Salad

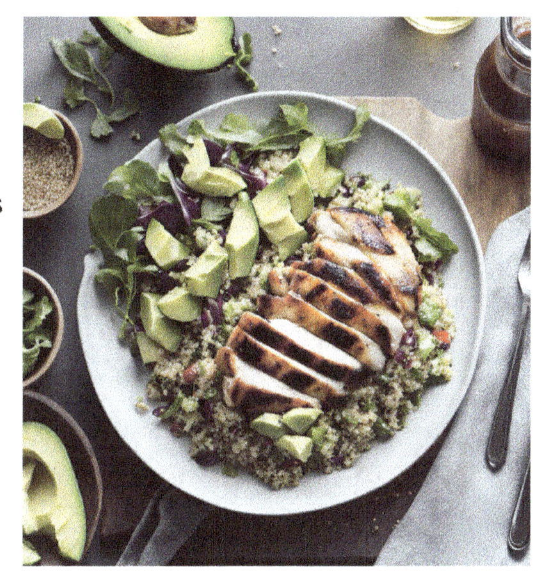

Preparation Time

Total: 30 minutes

Nutrition (per serving)

Calories: 350
Protein: 30g
Carbohydrates: 28g
Fiber: 8g
Fat: 15g

ingredients

For the Chicken:

- 2 boneless, skinless chicken breasts
- 1 tablespoon olive oil
- 1 teaspoon garlic powder
- 1 teaspoon paprika
- Salt and pepper to taste

For the Salad:

- 1 cup quinoa, cooked
- 1 avocado, diced
- 1 cup cherry tomatoes, halved
- 1/4 cup red onion, finely chopped
- 1/4 cup fresh cilantro, chopped
- 2 tablespoons lime juice
- 1 tablespoon olive oil
- Salt and pepper to taste

Instructions

1. Preheat your grill to mediumhigh heat.
2. Rub the chicken breasts with olive oil, garlic powder, paprika, salt, and pepper.
3. Grill the chicken for 68 minutes on each side or until fully cooked.
4. Let the chicken rest for a few minutes before slicing.
5. combine the cooked quinoa, diced avocado, cherry tomatoes, red onion, and cilantro in a large bowl.
6. whisk together the lime juice, olive oil, salt, and pepper in a small bowl.
7. Pour the dressing over the quinoa salad and toss to combine.
8. Serve the grilled chicken slices over the quinoa and avocado salad.

This Baked Salmon with Steamed Broccoli is a simple yet elegant dish full of flavour and nutrition. The tender, flaky salmon paired with perfectly steamed broccoli makes a delightful, zeropoint meal perfect for any occasion.

Baked Salmon with Steamed Broccoli

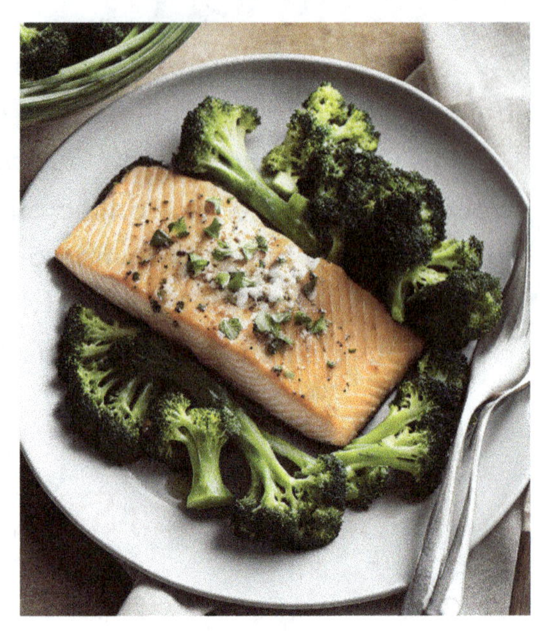

Preparation Time 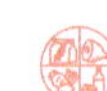

Total: 25 minutes

Nutrition (per serving)

Calories: 250
Protein: 28g
Carbohydrates: 8g
Fiber: 4g
Fat: 12g

ingredients

2 salmon fillets

1 tablespoon olive oil

2 garlic cloves, minced

1 lemon, sliced

Salt and pepper to taste

1 bunch broccoli, cut into florets

Instructions

1. Preheat your oven to 400°F (200°C).
2. Place the salmon fillets on a baking sheet lined with parchment paper.
3. Drizzle with olive oil, sprinkle with minced garlic, and season with salt and pepper.
4. Arrange lemon slices on top of the salmon fillets.
5. Bake for 1520 minutes until the salmon is cooked through and flakes easily with a fork.
6. While the salmon is baking, steam the broccoli florets in a steamer basket over boiling water for 57 minutes, until tender.
7. Serve the baked salmon with steamed broccoli on the side.

About the recipe

Savor the classic flavors of Eggplant Parmesan more healthily. This dish features layers of tender eggplant slices, rich tomato sauce, and melted cheese, all baked to perfection for a delicious, guiltfree meal.

Eggplant Parmesan

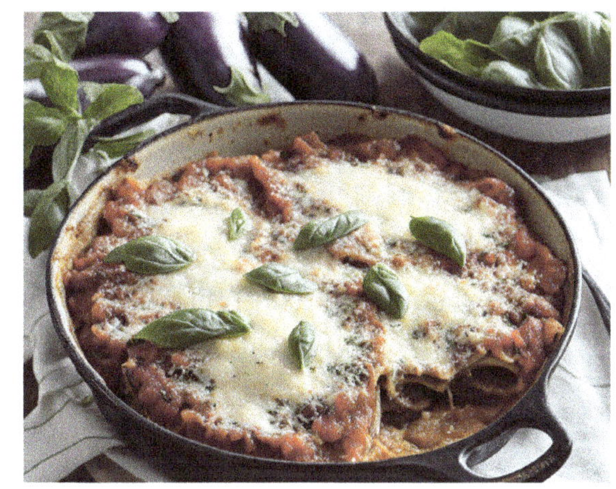

Preparation Time

Total: 50 minutes

Nutrition (per serving)

Calories: 220
Protein: 12g
Carbohydrates: 24g
Fiber: 7g
Fat: 10g

ingredients

- 1 large eggplant, sliced into 1/4inch rounds
- 1 cup whole wheat breadcrumbs
- 1/2 cup grated Parmesan cheese
- 2 eggs, beaten
- 2 cups marinara sauce
- 1 cup mozzarella cheese, shredded
- Fresh basil leaves for garnish

Instructions

1. Preheat your oven to 375°F (190°C).

2. Dip each eggplant slice into the beaten eggs, then coat with the breadcrumbs mixed with Parmesan cheese.

3. Place the coated eggplant slices on a baking sheet lined with parchment paper.

4. Bake for 20 minutes, flipping halfway through, until golden brown.

5. Spread a thin layer of marinara sauce in a baking dish.

6. Arrange a layer of baked eggplant slices on top of the Sauce.

7. Add another layer of marinara sauce and sprinkle with mozzarella cheese.

8. Repeat the layers, finishing with a layer of Sauce and cheese on top.

9. Bake for 2025 minutes until the cheese is melted and bubbly. Garnish with fresh basil leaves before serving.

Enjoy a lowcarb twist on a classic favorite with Spaghetti Squash and Meatballs. The tender strands of spaghetti squash perfectly complement the savory meatballs and marinara sauce, making this dish delicious and nutritious.

Spaghetti Squash and Meatballs

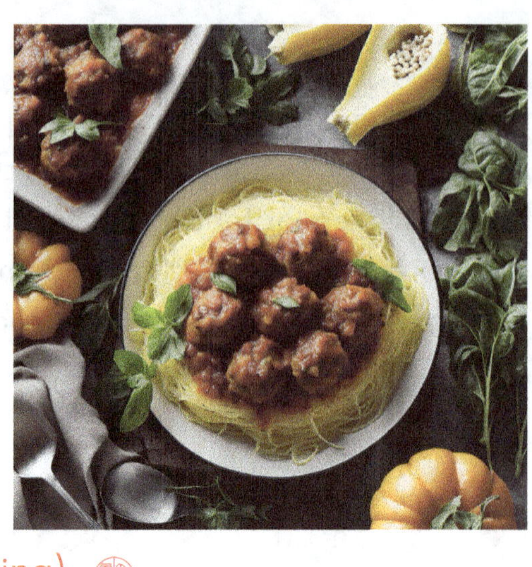

Preparation Time 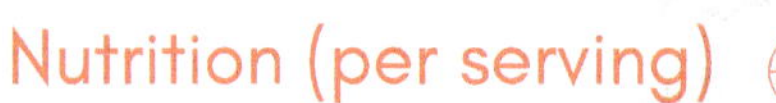

Total: 60 minutes

Nutrition (per serving)

Calories: 300
Protein: 24g
Carbohydrates: 24g
Fiber: 6g
Fat: 12g

ingredients

- 1 large spaghetti squash
- 1 lb lean ground turkey
- 1/4 cup grated Parmesan cheese
- 1/4 cup whole wheat breadcrumbs
- 1 egg
- 2 garlic cloves, minced
- 1 teaspoon dried oregano
- 2 cups marinara sauce
- Fresh basil leaves for garnish
- Salt and pepper to taste

Instructions

1. Preheat your oven to 400°F (200°C).
2. Cut the spaghetti squash in half lengthwise and remove the seeds.
3. Place the squash halves cut side down on a baking sheet and roast for 40 minutes or until tender.
4. combine the ground turkey, Parmesan cheese, breadcrumbs, egg, minced garlic, dried oregano, salt, and pepper in a bowl. Mix well and form into meatballs.
5. Place the meatballs on a baking sheet lined with parchment paper and bake for 20 minutes, until cooked.
6. Heat the marinara sauce in a saucepan over medium heat.
7. Use a fork to scrape the spaghetti squash strands into a serving bowl.
8. Top with meatballs and marinara sauce.
9. Garnish with fresh basil leaves before serving.

About the recipe

Grilled Portobello Mushrooms with Herbed Quinoa is a flavorful, satisfying dish perfect for a healthy meal. The meaty texture of the mushrooms paired with the nutty, herby quinoa makes this a delicious

Grilled Portobello Mushrooms with Herbed Quinoa

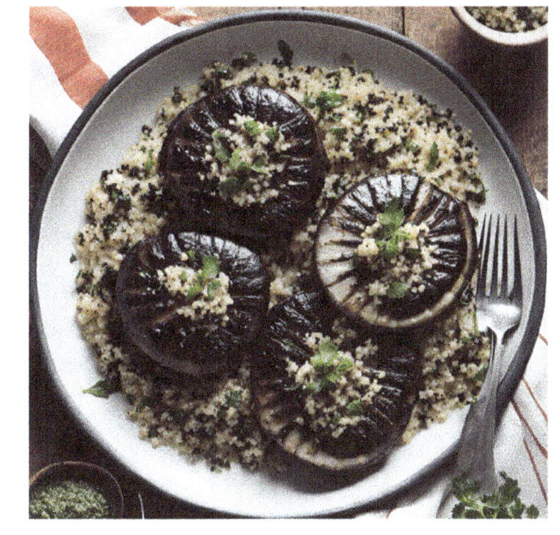

Preparation Time

Total: 30 minutes

Nutrition (per serving)

Calories: 220
Protein: 7g
Carbohydrates: 28g
Fiber: 5g
Fat: 10g

ingredients

For the Mushrooms:

- 4 large Portobello mushrooms, stems removed
- 2 tablespoons olive oil
- 2 garlic cloves, minced
- 1 tablespoon balsamic vinegar
- Salt and pepper to taste

For the Quinoa:

- 1 cup quinoa, rinsed
- 2 cups vegetable broth
- 1/4 cup fresh parsley, chopped
- 1/4 cup fresh cilantro, chopped
- 1 tablespoon lemon juice
- Salt and pepper to taste

Instructions

1. Preheat your grill to mediumhigh heat.
2. whisk together the olive oil, minced garlic, balsamic vinegar, salt, and pepper in a small bowl.
3. Brush the Portobello mushrooms with the marinade.
4. Grill the mushrooms on each side for 57 minutes until tender and slightly charred.
5. While the mushrooms are grilling, bring the vegetable broth to a boil in a saucepan.
6. Add the quinoa, reduce heat to low, cover, and simmer for 15 minutes until the quinoa is tender and the liquid is absorbed.
7. Fluff the quinoa with a fork and stir in the fresh parsley, cilantro, lemon juice, salt, and pepper.
8. Serve the grilled mushrooms over the herbed quinoa.

About the recipe

Spice your dinner with these flavorful Chicken Fajitas with Bell Peppers and Onion. Juicy chicken strips, vibrant bell peppers, and sweet onions combine in a sizzling, savoury, healthy and satisfying dish.

Chicken Fajitas with Bell Peppers and Onion

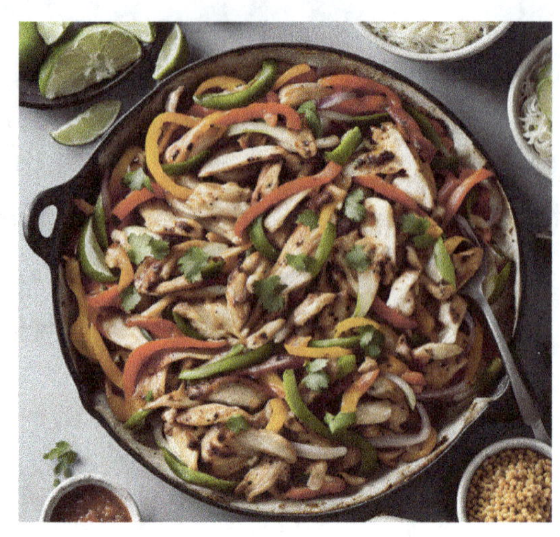

Preparation Time

Total: 25 minutes

Nutrition (per serving)

Calories: 250
Protein: 28g
Carbohydrates: 12g
Fiber: 3g
Fat: 10g

ingredients

- 2 boneless, skinless chicken breasts sliced into thin strips
- 1 red bell pepper, sliced
- 1 green bell pepper, sliced
- 1 yellow bell pepper, sliced
- 1 large onion, sliced
- 2 tablespoons olive oil
- 2 garlic cloves, minced
- 1 teaspoon chili powder
- 1 teaspoon cumin
- 1 teaspoon paprika
- Salt and pepper to taste
- Whole wheat tortillas (optional)
- Fresh cilantro, chopped (for garnish)
- Lime wedges (for serving)

Instructions

1. In a large bowl, combine the olive oil, minced garlic, chilli powder, cumin, paprika, salt, and pepper. Add the chicken strips and toss to coat.

2. Heat a large skillet over mediumhigh heat. Add the chicken and cook for 57 minutes until cooked through and lightly browned. Remove from the skillet and set aside.

3. In the same skillet, add the bell peppers and onion. Cook for 57 minutes until tender and slightly charred.

4. Return the chicken to the skillet and stir to combine with the vegetables. Cook for another 23 minutes until heated through.

5. Serve the fajita mixture in whole wheat tortillas (if using), garnished with fresh cilantro and lime wedges.

About the recipe

This Baked Cod with Ratatouille is a light and flavorful dish that combines tender, flaky cod with a medley of roasted vegetables. It's a healthy, colourful meal perfect for any night of the week.

Baked Cod with Ratatouille

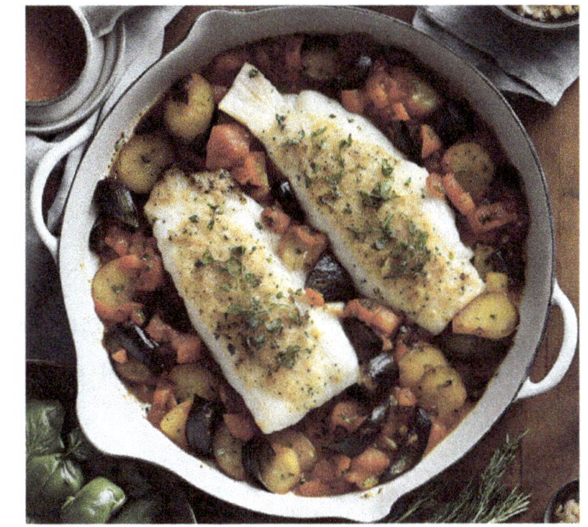

Preparation Time

Total: 45 minutes

Nutrition (per serving)

Calories: 220
Protein: 28g
Carbohydrates: 14g
Fiber: 5g
Fat: 8g

ingredients

For the Cod:

- 4 cod fillets
- 2 tablespoons olive oil
- 1 lemon, sliced
- Salt and pepper to taste

For the Ratatouille:

- 1 eggplant, diced
- 1 zucchini, diced
- 1 red bell pepper, diced
- 1 yellow bell pepper, diced
- 1 onion, diced
- 2 garlic cloves, minced
- 2 cups cherry tomatoes, halved
- 2 tablespoons olive oil
- 1 teaspoon dried thyme
- 1 teaspoon dried basil
- Salt and pepper to taste

Instructions

1. Preheat your oven to 400°F (200°C).
2. toss the diced eggplant, zucchini, bell peppers, onion, garlic, and cherry tomatoes with olive oil, thyme, basil, salt, and pepper in a large baking dish.
3. Bake the vegetables for 20 minutes.
4. Remove the baking dish from the oven and place the cod fillets on the vegetables. Drizzle with olive oil and season with salt and pepper. Top each fillet with lemon slices.
5. Return to the oven and bake for 1520 minutes until the cod is cooked and flakes easily with a fork.
6. Serve hot, with the ratatouille as a flavorful base for the cod.

Ditch the traditional bun and enjoy a healthy twist with this Veggie Burger with Sweet Potato Bun. Packed with flavour and nutrients, this dish is a delicious way to enjoy a burger while keeping it light and nutritious.

Veggie Burger with Sweet Potato Bun

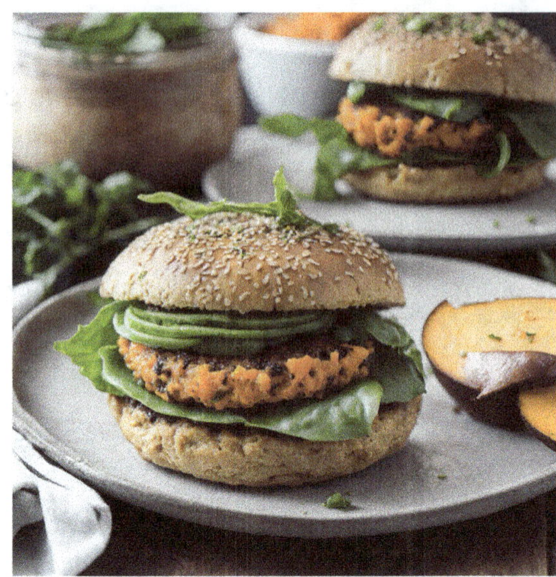

Preparation Time 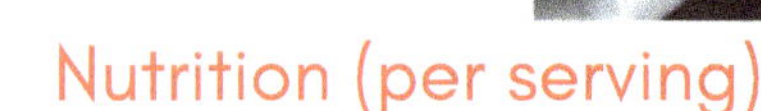

Total: 40 minutes

Nutrition (per serving)

Calories: 300
Protein: 10g
Carbohydrates: 40g
Fiber: 10g
Fat: 12g

ingredients

For the Veggie Burger:
- 1 can black beans, drained and rinsed
- 1 cup cooked quinoa
- 1/2 cup breadcrumbs
- 1 small onion, finely chopped
- 2 garlic cloves, minced
- 1 teaspoon cumin
- 1 teaspoon paprika
- Salt and pepper to taste
- 1 egg

For the Sweet Potato Bun:
- 2 large sweet potatoes, sliced into 1/2inch rounds
- 1 tablespoon olive oil
- Salt and pepper to taste

Instructions

1. Preheat your oven to 400°F (200°C).

2. In a large bowl, mash the black beans until mostly smooth. Add the cooked quinoa, breadcrumbs, chopped onion, minced garlic, cumin, paprika, salt, pepper, and egg. Mix until well combined.

3. Form the mixture into patties and place them on a baking sheet lined with parchment paper. Bake for 20 minutes, flipping halfway through, until firm and golden brown.

4. While the patties are baking, prepare the sweet potato buns. Toss the sweet potato rounds with olive oil, salt, and

- For the Veggie Burger:
- 1 can black beans, drained and rinsed
- 1 cup cooked quinoa
- 1/2 cup breadcrumbs
- 1 small onion, finely chopped
- 2 garlic cloves, minced
- 1 teaspoon cumin
- 1 teaspoon paprika
- Salt and pepper to taste

pepper. Arrange them on another baking sheet and bake for 1520 minutes, flipping halfway through, until tender and slightly crispy.

5. Assemble the veggie burgers by placing each patty between two sweet potato rounds. Top with avocado, lettuce, tomato, and red onion slices.

6. Serve immediately and enjoy!

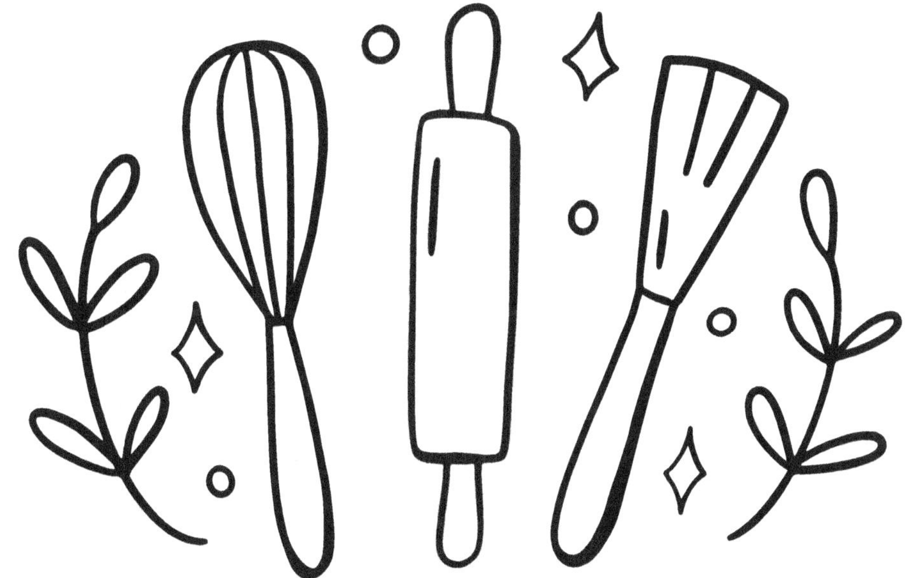

Warm, comforting, and with a zingy twist, this Butternut Squash Soup with a Twist of Ginger is the perfect cosy meal. The sweetness of the squash paired with the spicy ginger creates a delightful blend of flavors.

Butternut Squash Soup with a Twist of Ginger

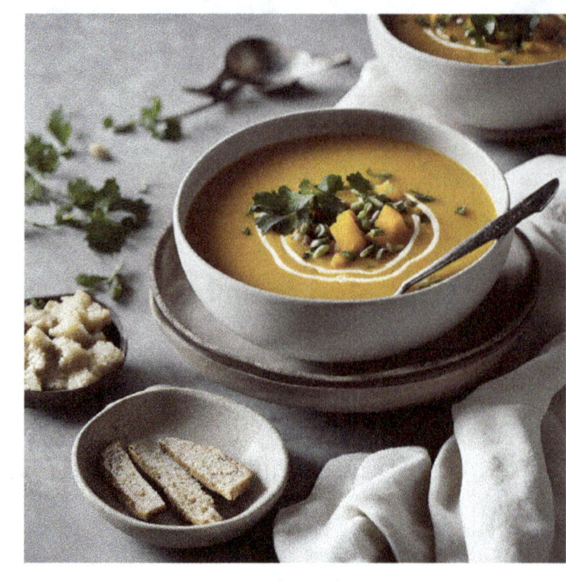

Preparation Time

Total: 35 minutes

Nutrition (per serving)

Calories: 150
Protein: 3g
Carbohydrates: 30g
Fiber: 5g
Fat: 4g

ingredients

- 1 large butternut squash, peeled and cubed
- 1 onion, chopped
- 2 garlic cloves, minced
- 1 tablespoon olive oil
- 1 tablespoon fresh ginger, grated
- 4 cups vegetable broth
- Salt and pepper to taste
- Fresh cilantro for garnish (optional)

Instructions

1. heat the olive oil over medium heat in a large pot.

2. Add the chopped onion and cook until softened about 5 minutes.

3. Add the minced garlic and grated ginger, cooking for another minute.

4. Stir in the cubed butternut squash and vegetable broth. Bring to a boil, reduce the heat and simmer for 2025 minutes until the squash is tender.

5. Use an immersion blender to blend the soup until smooth.

6. Season with salt and pepper to taste.

7. Serve hot, garnished with fresh cilantro if desired.

About the recipe

This Quinoa Salad with Roasted Vegetables is a vibrant and nutritious dish that is perfect as a side or a light main course. Packed with colourful roasted vegetables and nutty quinoa, it's a delicious and healthy option for any meal.

Quinoa Salad with Roasted Vegetables

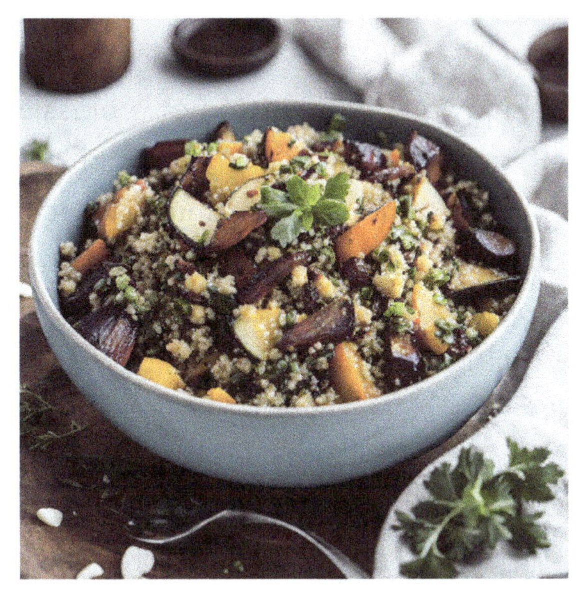

Preparation Time 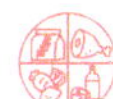

Total: 35 minutes

Nutrition (per serving)

Calories: 200
Protein: 6g
Carbohydrates: 28g
Fiber: 6g
Fat: 8g

ingredients

- 1 cup quinoa, cooked
- 1 red bell pepper, diced
- 1 yellow bell pepper, diced
- 1 zucchini, diced
- 1 red onion, diced
- 2 tablespoons olive oil
- 1 teaspoon dried oregano
- Salt and pepper to taste
- 1/4 cup fresh parsley, chopped
- 2 tablespoons lemon juice

Instructions

1. Preheat your oven to 425°F (220°C).
2. On a large baking sheet, toss the diced bell peppers, zucchini, red onion with olive oil, dried oregano, salt, and pepper.
3. Roast the vegetables for 2025 minutes until tender and slightly charred.
4. combine the cooked quinoa, roasted vegetables, chopped parsley, and lemon juice in a large bowl.
5. Toss to combine and season with additional salt and pepper if needed.
6. Serve warm or at room temperature.

About the recipe

Enjoy a lighter version of a classic comfort food with this Zucchini Lasagna. Layers of thinly sliced zucchini, rich tomato sauce, and melted cheese make this dish a delightful, guiltfree option for any night of the week.

Zucchini Lasagna

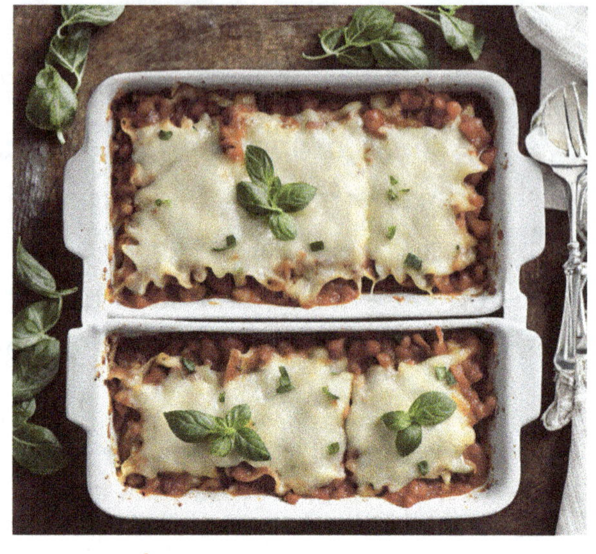

Preparation Time

Total: 45 minutes

Nutrition (per serving)

Calories: 250
Protein: 15g
Carbohydrates: 12g
Fiber: 3g
Fat: 16g

ingredients

- 3 large zucchinis, sliced lengthwise into thin strips
- 2 cups marinara sauce
- 1 cup ricotta cheese
- 1/2 cup grated Parmesan cheese
- 1 cup shredded mozzarella cheese
- 1 egg
- 2 garlic cloves, minced
- 1 tablespoon olive oil
- Salt and pepper to taste
- Fresh basil leaves for garnish

Instructions

1. Preheat your oven to 375°F (190°C).
2. Combine the ricotta cheese, grated Parmesan cheese, egg, minced garlic, salt, and pepper in a bowl.
3. Spread a thin layer of marinara sauce in a baking dish.
4. Arrange a layer of zucchini slices over the Sauce.
5. Spread a layer of the ricotta mixture over the zucchini, followed by a layer of marinara sauce.
6. Repeat the layers, finishing with a layer of marinara sauce and shredded mozzarella cheese on top.
7. Bake for 3035 minutes until the cheese is melted and bubbly.
8. Garnish with fresh basil leaves before serving.

About the recipe

This Cauliflower Fried Rice is a healthy, zero point alternative without skimping on flavor. Packed with vegetables and bursting with the savory taste you love, it's a quick and satisfying meal perfect for any night of the week.

Cauliflower Fried Rice

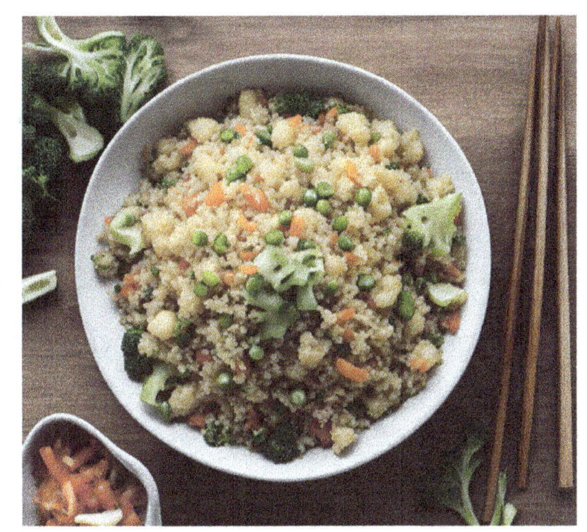

Preparation Time 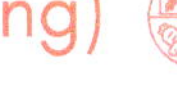

Total: 45 minutes

Nutrition (per serving)

Calories: 250
Protein: 15g
Carbohydrates: 12g
Fiber: 3g
Fat: 16g

ingredients

- 1 large head of cauliflower, riced
- 1 tablespoon olive oil
- 1 onion, diced
- 2 garlic cloves, minced
- 1 cup frozen peas and carrots
- 2 eggs, beaten
- 3 tablespoons soy sauce (low sodium)
- 2 green onions, sliced
- Salt and pepper to taste

Instructions

1. In a food processor, pulse the cauliflower florets until they resemble rice grains.
2. Heat olive oil in a large skillet over medium heat. Add the diced onion and cook until softened about 5 minutes.
3. Add the minced garlic and cook for another minute.
4. Stir in the peas and carrots, cooking until heated, about 3 minutes.
5. Push the vegetables to one side of the skillet and pour the beaten eggs into the space. Scramble the eggs until fully cooked, then mix with the vegetables.
6. Add the cauliflower rice to the skillet and cook for 57 minutes, until tender.
7. Stir in the soy sauce and season with salt and pepper.
8. Garnish with sliced green onions and serve

Warm up with a hearty bowl of Vegetable and Bean Chili. This zeropoint dish is packed with various vegetables and beans, creating a deliciously rich and satisfying meal perfect for cosy nights.

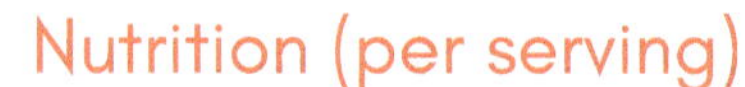

Vegetable and Bean Chili

Preparation Time

Total: 45 minutes

Nutrition (per serving)

Calories: 200
Protein: 10g
Carbohydrates: 35g
Fiber: 12g
Fat: 4g

ingredients

- 1 tablespoon olive oil
- 1 onion, chopped
- 3 garlic cloves, minced
- 2 bell peppers, diced
- 2 zucchinis, diced
- 1 can black beans, drained and rinsed
- 1 can kidney beans, drained and rinsed
- 1 can diced tomatoes
- 2 cups vegetable broth
- 2 tablespoons chili powder
- 1 teaspoon cumin
- 1 teaspoon paprika
- Salt and pepper to taste

Instructions

1. Heat olive oil in a large pot over medium heat. Add the chopped onion and cook until softened about 5 minutes.
2. Add the minced garlic and cook for another minute.
3. Stir in the diced bell peppers and zucchinis, cooking until tender, about 5 minutes.
4. Add the black beans, kidney beans, diced tomatoes, and vegetable broth.
5. Stir in the chilli powder, cumin, and paprika. Bring to a boil, then reduce heat and simmer for 30 minutes.
6. Season with salt and pepper to taste.
7. Serve hot, garnished with your favourite chilli toppings if desired.

These Turkey and Spinach Meatballs in Tomato Sauce are a delightful, protein packed, healthy and flavorful dish. The combination of lean turkey and fresh spinach creates tender meatballs simmered in a rich tomato sauce for a comforting meal.

Turkey and Spinach Meatballs in Tomato Sauce

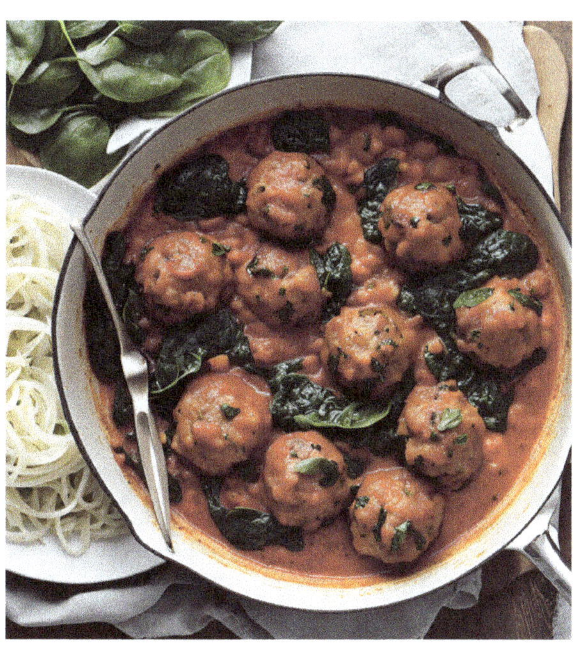

Preparation Time

Total: 45 minutes

Nutrition (per serving)

Calories: 250
Protein: 20g
Carbohydrates: 10g
Fiber: 3g
Fat: 12g

ingredients

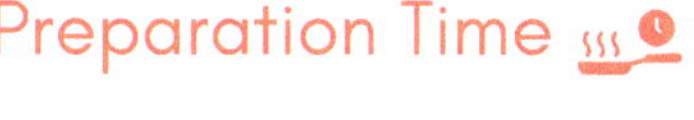

For the Meatballs:

- 1 lb lean ground turkey
- 1 cup fresh spinach, chopped
- 1/4 cup grated Parmesan cheese
- 1/4 cup whole wheat breadcrumbs
- 1 egg
- 2 garlic cloves, minced
- Salt and pepper to taste

For the Tomato Sauce:

- 1 tablespoon olive oil
- 1 onion, chopped

Instructions

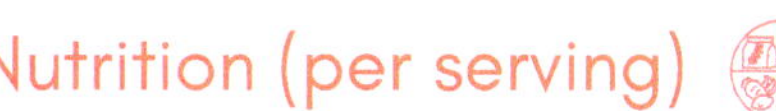

1. Preheat the oven to 375°F (190°C). Combine the ground turkey, chopped spinach, Parmesan cheese, breadcrumbs, egg, minced garlic, salt, and pepper in a large bowl. Mix until well combined.

2. Form the mixture into meatballs and place them on a baking sheet lined with parchment paper. Bake for 20 minutes until cooked through.

3. While the meatballs are baking, prepare the tomato sauce. Heat olive oil in a large skillet over medium heat. Add the chopped onion and cook until softened about 5 minutes.

4. Add the minced garlic and cook for another minute.

- 2 garlic cloves, minced
- 1 can crushed tomatoes
- 1 teaspoon dried oregano
- Salt and pepper to taste
- Fresh basil leaves for garnish

5. Stir in the crushed tomatoes and dried oregano. Bring to a simmer and cook for 15 minutes—season with salt and pepper.

6. Add the baked meatballs to the tomato sauce and simmer for 10 minutes.

7. Serve hot, garnished with fresh basil leaves.

Stuffed Acorn Squash is a delightful, hearty dish perfect for fall or whenever you crave something warm and comforting. The sweet acorn squash is filled with a savory mixture of vegetables and quinoa, creating an ideal balance of flavors.

Stuffed Acorn Squash

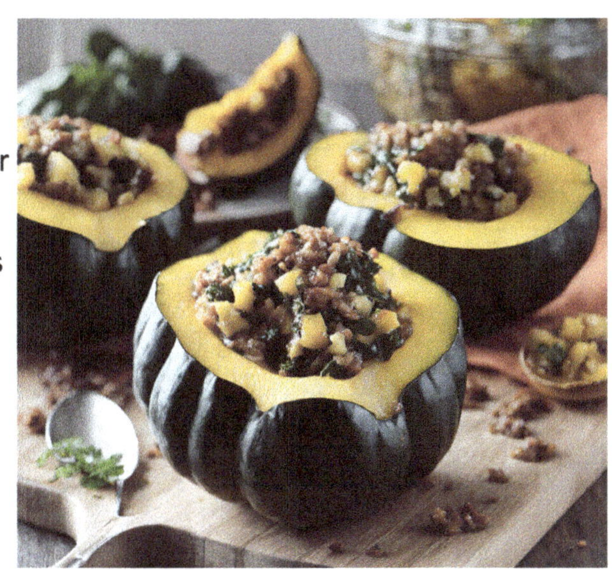

Preparation Time

Total: 45 minutes

Nutrition (per serving)

Calories: 200
Protein: 8g
Carbohydrates: 40g
Fiber: 8g
Fat: 6g

ingredients

- 2 acorn squashes, halved and seeded
- 1 cup quinoa, cooked
- 1 bell pepper, diced
- 1 onion, diced
- 2 garlic cloves, minced
- 1 cup black beans, drained and rinsed
- 1 teaspoon cumin
- 1 teaspoon paprika
- 2 tablespoons olive oil
- Salt and pepper to taste
- Fresh parsley for garnish

Instructions

1. Preheat your oven to 400°F (200°C). Place the acorn squash halves cut side down on a baking sheet and roast for 2530 minutes, until tender.
2. While the squash is roasting, heat olive oil in a large skillet over medium heat. Add the diced onion and bell pepper, cooking until softened, about 5 minutes.
3. Add the minced garlic and cook for another minute.
4. Stir in the cooked quinoa, black beans, cumin, and paprika. Cook for another 5 minutes until heated through, then season with salt and pepper.
5. Remove the squash from the oven and flip them cut side up. Fill each half with the quinoa mixture.
6. Return to the oven and bake for an additional 10 minutes.
7. Garnish with fresh parsley before serving.

About the recipe

This Shrimp and Asparagus Stir Fry is a quick and easy dish full of flavor and nutrition. Juicy shrimp and tender asparagus are stir-fried with garlic and a touch of soy sauce for a light, delicious meal for busy nights.

Shrimp and Asparagus Stir Fry

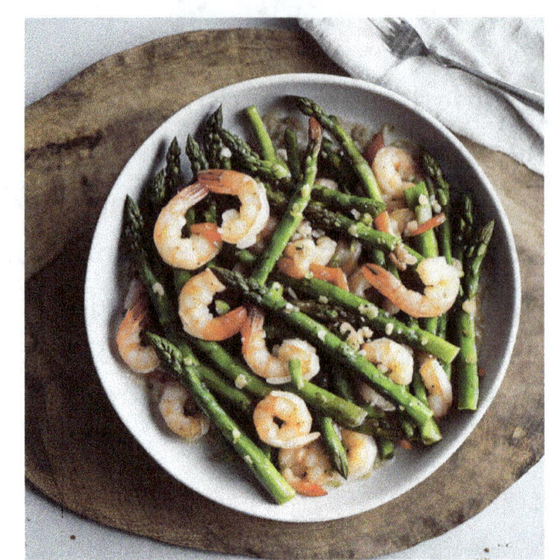

Preparation Time

Total: 20 minutes

Nutrition (per serving)

Calories: 200
Protein: 25g
Carbohydrates: 8g
Fiber: 3g
Fat: 8g

ingredients

- 1 lb shrimp, peeled and deveined
- 1 bunch asparagus, trimmed and cut into 2inch pieces
- 2 tablespoons olive oil
- 3 garlic cloves, minced
- 2 tablespoons soy sauce (low sodium)
- 1 tablespoon lemon juice
- Salt and pepper to taste
- Fresh parsley for garnish

Instructions

1. Heat olive oil in a large skillet or wok over medium high heat. Add the minced garlic and cook for 1 minute until fragrant.
2. Add the shrimp to the skillet and cook for 23 minutes until pink and opaque. Remove the shrimp from the skillet and set aside.
3. In the same skillet, add the asparagus and cook for 57 minutes until tender crisp.
4. Return the shrimp to the skillet and stir in the soy sauce and lemon juice. Cook for another 2 minutes until heated through.
5. Season with salt and pepper to taste.
6. Serve hot, garnished with fresh parsley.

About the recipe

Cozy up with a bowl of this hearty Lentil and Sweet Potato Stew. Packed with nutrients and flavor, this stew is a comforting, zero point meal perfect for chilly days or when you need a little extra warmth. The combination of tender lentils and sweet potatoes makes every spoonful satisfying and delicious.

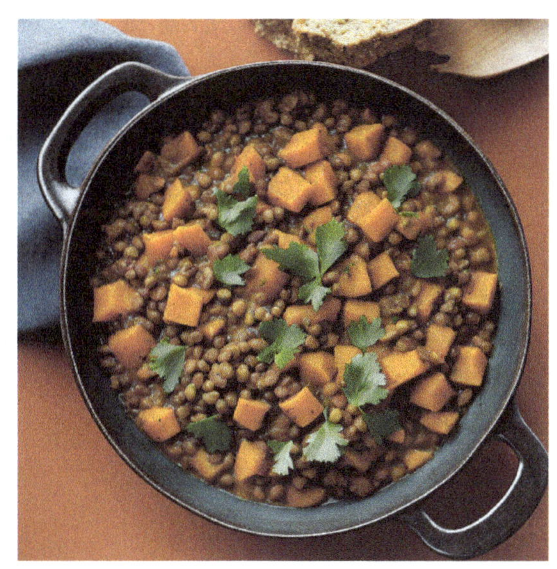

Lentil and Sweet Potato Stew

Preparation Time 

Total: 45 minutes

Nutrition (per serving)

Calories: 250
Protein: 12g
Carbohydrates: 40g
Fiber: 12g
Fat: 6g

ingredients

- 1 tablespoon olive oil
- 1 onion, chopped
- 3 garlic cloves, minced
- 2 sweet potatoes, peeled and diced
- 1 cup dried lentils, rinsed
- 4 cups vegetable broth
- 1 can diced tomatoes
- 2 teaspoons cumin
- 1 teaspoon smoked paprika
- Salt and pepper to taste
- Fresh cilantro for garnish

Instructions

1. Heat the olive oil in a large pot over medium heat. Add the chopped onion and cook until softened about 5 minutes.
2. Add the minced garlic and cook for another minute until fragrant.
3. Stir in the diced sweet potatoes, lentils, vegetable broth, tomatoes, cumin, and smoked paprika.
4. Bring to a boil, then reduce the heat and simmer for 3035 minutes until the lentils and sweet potatoes are tender.
5. Season with salt and pepper to taste.
6. Serve hot, garnished with fresh cilantro.

These Stuffed Peppers with Ground Turkey and Quinoa are a delightful and nutritious meal perfect for any day of the week. The bell peppers are filled with a savory mixture of lean turkey, quinoa, and vegetables, making for a satisfying and healthy dish.

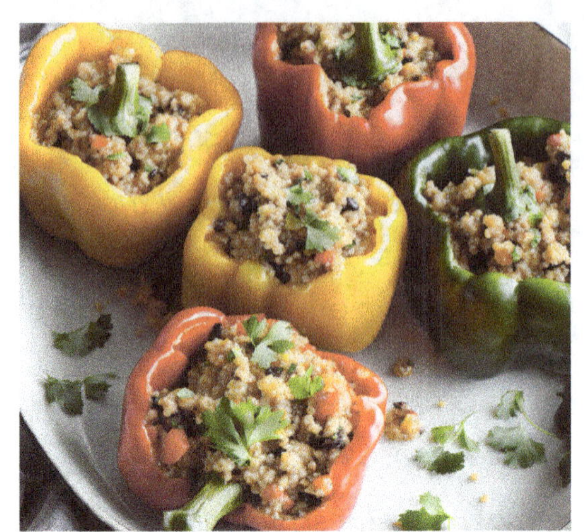

Stuffed Peppers with Ground Turkey and Quinoa

Preparation Time 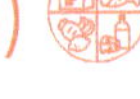

Total: 45 minutes

Nutrition (per serving)

Calories: 300
Protein: 25g
Carbohydrates: 30g
Fiber: 7g
Fat: 8g

ingredients

- 4 large bell peppers, tops cut off and seeds removed
- 1 lb ground turkey
- 1 cup cooked quinoa
- 1 onion, diced
- 2 garlic cloves, minced
- 1 can diced tomatoes
- 1 teaspoon cumin
- 1 teaspoon paprika
- Salt and pepper to taste
- 1/4 cup shredded mozzarella cheese (optional)

Instructions

1. Preheat your oven to 375°F (190°C).
2. In a large skillet, cook the ground turkey over medium heat until browned, about 57 minutes.
3. Add the diced onion and cook until softened about 5 minutes. Add the minced garlic and cook for another minute.
4. Stir in the cooked quinoa, diced tomatoes, cumin, paprika, salt, and pepper. Cook for another 5 minutes until heated through.
5. Stuff each bell pepper with the turkey and quinoa mixture and place them in a baking dish.
6. If using, sprinkle shredded mozzarella cheese on top of each stuffed pepper.
7. Cover the baking dish with foil and bake for 2530 minutes until the peppers are tender.
8. Serve hot and enjoy!

About the recipe

Elevate your dinner with this pan eared tuna with Avocado Salsa. The tuna steaks are perfectly seared to a tender finish and topped with fresh, zesty avocado salsa. This dish is light, flavorful, and packed with healthy fats and proteins.

Pan seared tuna with Avocado Salsa

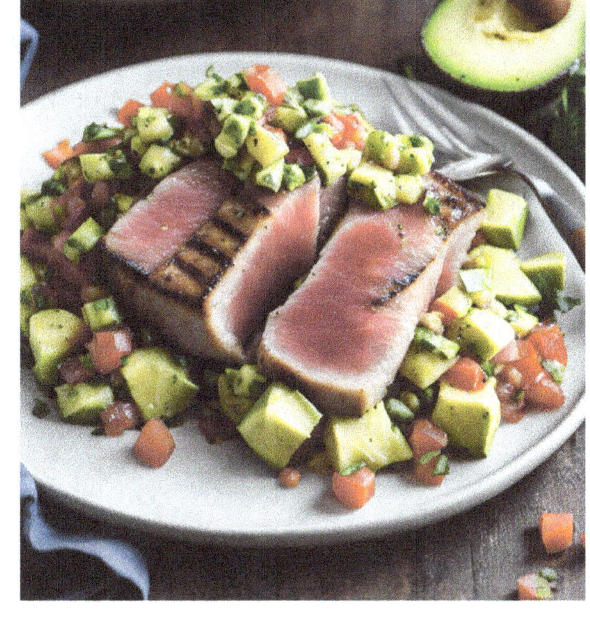

Preparation Time

Total: 15 minutes

Nutrition (per serving)

Calories: 350
Protein: 30g
Carbohydrates: 12g
Fiber: 8g
Fat: 20g

ingredients

For the Tuna:

- 2 tuna steaks
- 1 tablespoon olive oil
- Salt and pepper to taste
- 1 teaspoon sesame seeds (optional)

For the Avocado Salsa:

- 1 ripe avocado, diced
- 1/2 red onion, finely chopped
- 1 jalapeno, seeded and minced
- 1/4 cup fresh cilantro, chopped
- 2 tablespoons lime juice
- Salt and pepper to taste

Instructions

1. Season the tuna steaks with salt, pepper, and sesame seeds (if using).
2. Heat the olive oil in a skillet over medium high heat. Sear the tuna steaks for 23 minutes on each side for medium rare or until cooked to your desired level of doneness. Remove from the skillet and let rest.
3. While the tuna rests, prepare the avocado salsa. Combine the diced avocado, red onion, jalapeno, cilantro, lime juice, salt, and pepper in a bowl. Mix gently.
4. Serve the seared tuna steaks topped with the avocado salsa.

About the recipe

Roasted Vegetable and Hummus Wraps are a delicious, easy to make meal perfect for lunch or a light dinner. The roasted vegetables add an incredible depth of flavor, while the hummus provides a creamy, satisfying base.

Roasted Vegetable and Hummus Wraps

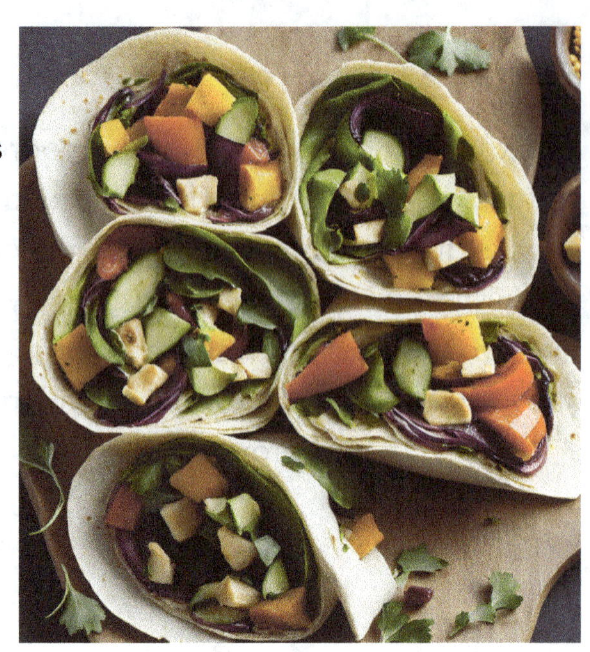

Preparation Time

Total: 30 minutes

Nutrition (per serving)

Calories: 250
Protein: 8g
Carbohydrates: 35g
Fiber: 10g
Fat: 10g

ingredients

- 1 zucchini, sliced
- 1 red bell pepper, sliced
- 1 yellow bell pepper, sliced
- 1 red onion, sliced
- 1 tablespoon olive oil
- 1 teaspoon dried oregano
- Salt and pepper to taste
- 4 whole wheat tortillas
- 1 cup hummus
- 2 cups fresh spinach leaves

Instructions

1. Preheat your oven to 400°F (200°C).
2. On a baking sheet, toss the sliced zucchini, bell peppers, red onion with olive oil, dried oregano, salt, and pepper.
3. Roast the vegetables for 2025 minutes until tender ad slightly charred.
4. Warm the whole wheat tortillas in the microwave or skillet for 30 seconds.
5. Spread a generous amount of hummus on each tortilla.
6. Top with roasted vegetables and fresh spinach leaves.
7. Roll up the wraps and serve immediately.

About the recipe

Indulge your sweet tooth without the guilt with these delightful Carrot Cake Bites. Packed with the flavors of a classic carrot cake but in a healthy, bite sized form, these treats are perfect for a quick snack or dessert.

Carrot Cake Bites

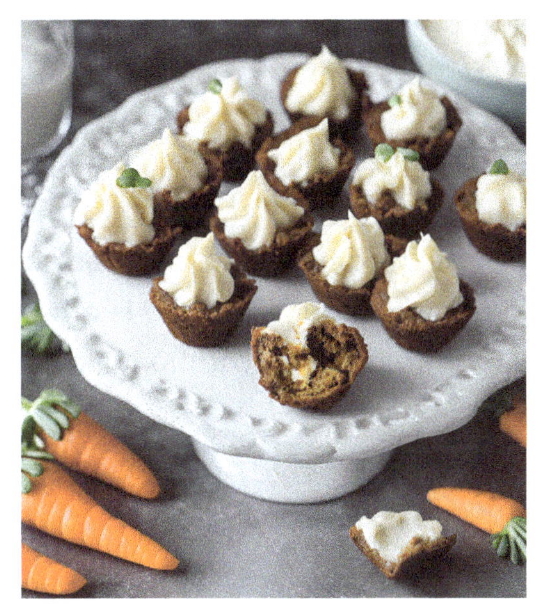

Preparation Time 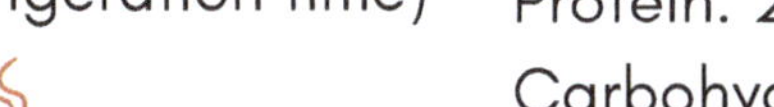

35 minutes
(including refrigeration time)

Nutrition (per serving)

Calories: 80
Protein: 2g
Carbohydrates: 12g
Fiber: 2g
Fat: 3g

ingredients

- 1 cup grated carrots
- 1/2 cup rolled oats
- 1/4 cup unsweetened applesauce
- 1/4 cup raisins
- 1/4 cup chopped walnuts
- 1 teaspoon cinnamon
- 1/2 teaspoon nutmeg
- 1/2 teaspoon vanilla extract

Instructions

1. Combine all the ingredients until well blended in a large bowl.

2. Form the mixture into small bite sized balls and place them on a baking sheet lined with parchment paper.

3. Refrigerate for at least 30 minutes to allow the bites to firm up.

4. Serve chilled and enjoy!

About the recipe

Satisfy your chocolate cravings with this creamy, guilt free Chocolate Banana Ice Cream. This frozen treat has just two ingredients and is a healthy alternative to traditional ice cream.

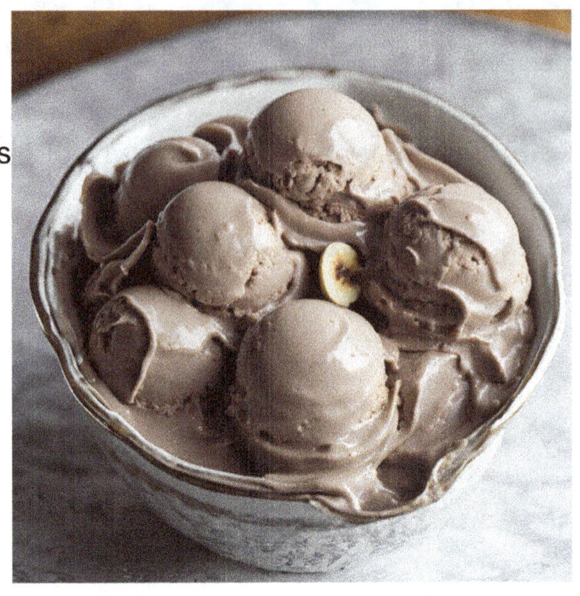

Chocolate Banana Ice Cream

Preparation Time
Total: 10 minutes
(plus optional additional freezing time)

Nutrition (per serving)

Calories: 120
Protein: 2g
Carbohydrates: 30g
Fiber: 4g
Fat: 1g

ingredients

- 4 ripe bananas, sliced and frozen
- 2 tablespoons unsweetened cocoa powder

Instructions

1. Place the frozen banana slices in a food processor and blend until smooth and creamy.

2. Add the unsweetened cocoa powder and blend until well combined.

3. Scoop the mixture into bowls and serve immediately for a soft serve consistency, or freeze for 12 hours for a firmer texture.

About the recipe

Enjoy the classic flavors of strawberry cheesecake in a convenient, no bake jar. This Strawberry Cheesecake Jar is a light, refreshing, and easy to make dessert. It's an ideal treat for a warm day or a sweet end to any meal.

Strawberry Cheesecake Jar

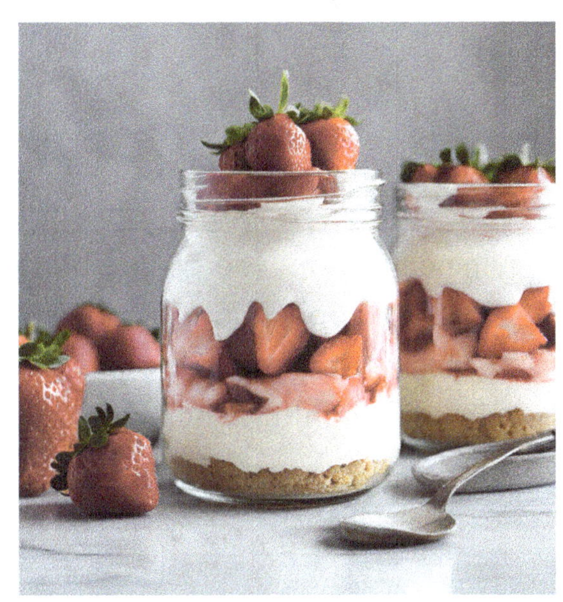

Preparation Time

Total: 35 minutes (including chilling time)

Nutrition (per serving)

Calories: 150
Protein: 10g
Carbohydrates: 25g
Fiber: 3g
Fat: 3g

ingredients

- 1 cup nonfat Greek yogurt
- 1/2 cup strawberries, chopped
- 1/4 cup granola
- 1 tablespoon honey
- 1 teaspoon vanilla extract

Instructions

1. Mix the Greek yoghurt, honey, and vanilla extract in a small bowl until well combined.

2. Layer the yoghurt mixture, chopped strawberries, and granola in a jar, starting with a layer of yoghurt.

3. Repeat the layers until the jar is full.

4. Chill in the refrigerator for at least 30 minutes before serving.

About the recipe

This Grilled Pineapple with Honey and Yogurt is a simple yet delectable summer dessert. The grilling brings out the pineapple's natural sweetness, while the honey and yogurt add a delightful creaminess.

Grilled Pineapple with Honey and Yogurt

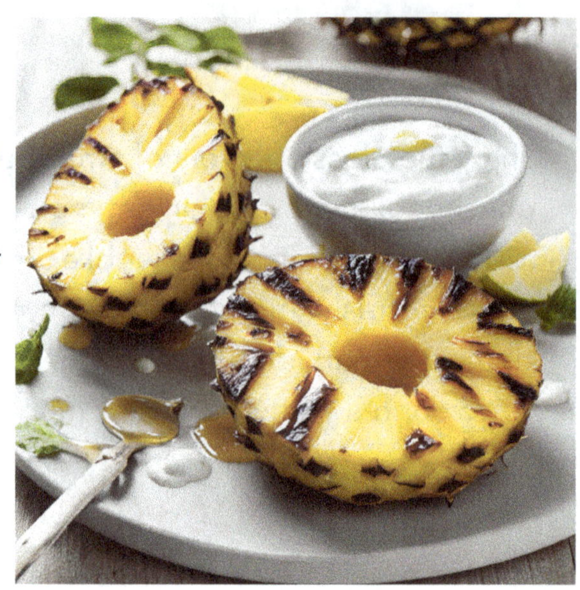

Preparation Time
Total: 15 minutes

Nutrition (per serving)

Calories: 100
Protein: 4g
Carbohydrates: 20g
Fiber: 2g
Fat: 1g

ingredients

- 1 pineapple, peeled, cored, and sliced
- 1 cup Greek yogurt
- 2 tablespoons honey
- Fresh mint leaves for garnish (optional)

Instructions

1. Preheat your grill to medium high heat.

2. Grill the pineapple slices on each side for 23 minutes until they are caramelized and have grill marks.

3. mix the Greek yoghurt and honey in a small bowl until well combined.

4. Serve the grilled pineapple slices topped with the honey yoghurt and garnish with fresh mint leaves if desired.

These Baked Apples with Cinnamon are a warm, comforting dessert perfect for a cosy night. The natural sweetness of the apples paired with the spicy cinnamon makes for a delightful treat that's healthy and delicious.

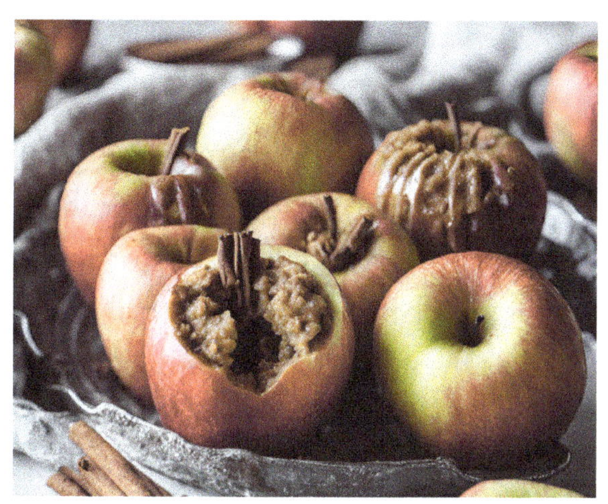

Baked Apples with Cinnamon

Preparation Time 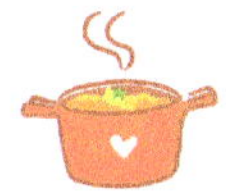
Total: 35 minutes

Nutrition (per serving)

Calories: 150
Protein: 2g
Carbohydrates: 30g
Fiber: 5g
Fat: 5g

ingredients

- 4 apples, cored
- 1/4 cup raisins
- 1/4 cup chopped walnuts
- 2 teaspoons cinnamon
- 1 tablespoon honey (optional)

Instructions

1. Preheat your oven to 375°F (190°C).

2. mix the raisins, chopped walnuts, and cinnamon in a small bowl.

3. Stuff each apple with the raisin and walnut mixture.

4. Place the stuffed apples in a baking dish and drizzle with honey if using.

5. Bake for 2530 minutes until the apples are tender.

6. Serve warm and enjoy!

About the recipe

Cool down with this refreshing Mixed Berry Sorbet, a delicious and healthy treat perfect for any time of the year. This sorbet is bursting with the natural sweetness of berries and is incredibly easy to make. It's a guilt free dessert that will satisfy your sweet cravings.

Mixed Berry Sorbet

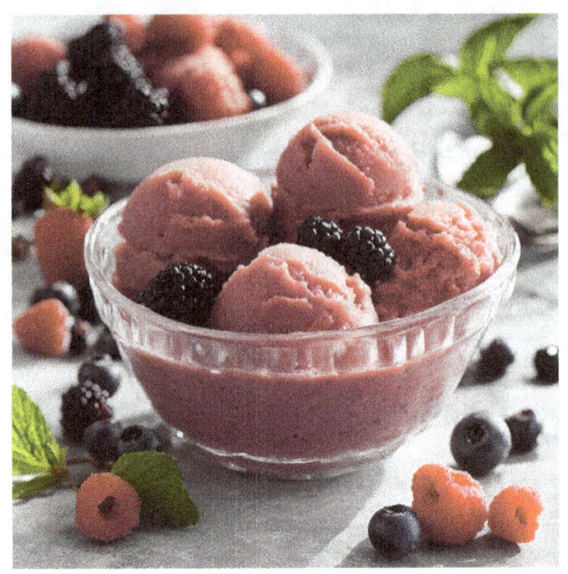

Preparation Time

Total: 2 hours (including freezing time)

Nutrition (per serving)

Calories: 80
Protein: 1g
Carbohydrates: 20g
Fiber: 6g
Fat: 0g

ingredients

- 4 cups mixed berries (strawberries, blueberries, raspberries, blackberries)
- 1/4 cup water
- 1 tablespoon lemon juice
- 1 tablespoon honey (optional)

Instructions

1. In a blender or food processor, combine the mixed berries, water, lemon juice, and honey (if using).

2. Blend until smooth.

3. Pour the mixture into a shallow container and freeze for 12 hours, stirring every 30 minutes until the sorbet is firm.

4. Scoop into bowls and serve immediately.

About the recipe

Indulge in these rich and creamy Dark Chocolate Avocado Truffles. Made with wholesome ingredients, these truffles are a decadent treat you can enjoy without guilt. Perfect for healthily satisfying your chocolate cravings!

Dark Chocolate Avocado Truffles

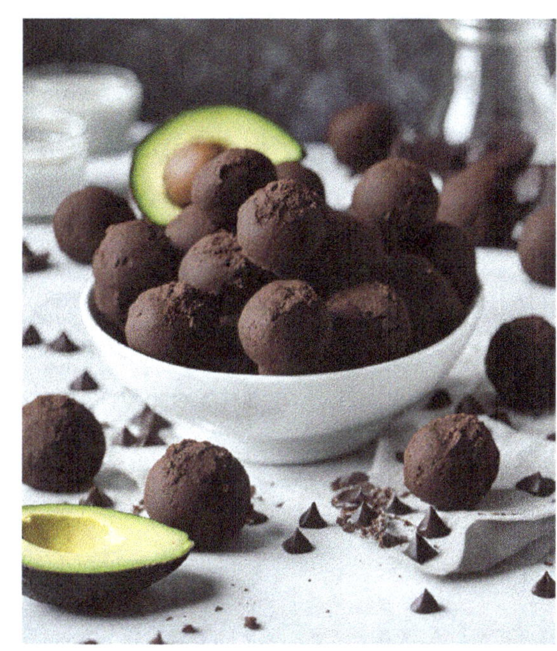

Preparation Time

Total: 45 minutes (including refrigeration time)

Nutrition (per serving)

Calories: 100
Protein: 1g
Carbohydrates: 10g
Fiber: 4g
Fat: 7g

ingredients

- 2 ripe avocados
- 1 cup dark chocolate chips
- 1 teaspoon vanilla extract
- 2 tablespoons cocoa powder (for rolling)

Instructions

1. Melt the dark chocolate chips in a microwave safe bowl or over a double boiler until smooth.

2. In a food processor, blend the avocados until creamy.

3. Add the melted chocolate and vanilla extract to the avocado and blend until well combined.

4. Refrigerate the mixture for about 30 minutes to firm up.

5. scoop out small portions and roll them into balls using a spoon.

6. Roll each ball in cocoa powder to coat.

7. Store in the refrigerator until ready to serve.

About the recipe

Enjoy a taste of the tropics with this Coconut and Lime Pinna Cotta. This creamy, dairy free dessert is infused with the refreshing flavors of coconut and lime, making it a light and delightful end to any meal.

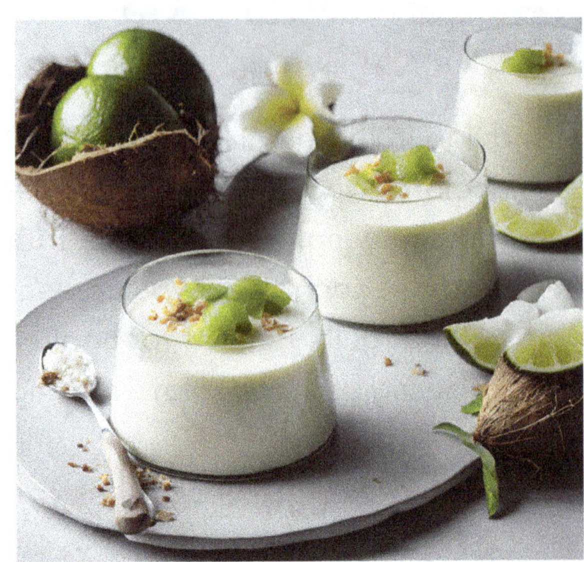

Coconut and Lime Panna Cotta

Preparation Time 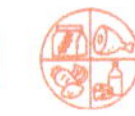

Total: 4 hours and 15 minutes (including refrigeration time)

Nutrition (per serving)

Calories: 150
Protein: 2g
Carbohydrates: 12g
Fiber: 2g
Fat: 12g

ingredients

- 1 cans (13.5 oz) fullfat coconut milk
- 2 tablespoons honey
- 1 teaspoon vanilla extract
- 1 tablespoon lime juice
- 1 teaspoon lime zest
- 1 packet (1 tablespoon) unflavored gelatin
- 1/4 cup cold water

Instructions

1. In a small bowl, sprinkle the gelatin over the cold water and let it sit for 5 minutes to bloom.

2. Combine the coconut milk, honey, and vanilla extract in a saucepan. Heat over medium heat until warm but not boiling.

3. Stir in the lime juice and lime zest.

4. Add the bloomed gelatin to the warm coconut milk mixture and stir until completely dissolved.

5. Pour the mixture into small ramekins or moulds and refrigerate for at least 4 hours or until set.

6. Serve chilled, garnished with extra lime zest if desired.

About the recipe

These colorful Fruit Kabobs with Yogurt Dip are a fun and healthy dessert for kids and adults alike. The creamy yoghurt dip adds a delicious touch to the fresh, juicy fruit, making it an irresistible treat.

Fruit Kabobs with Yogurt Dip

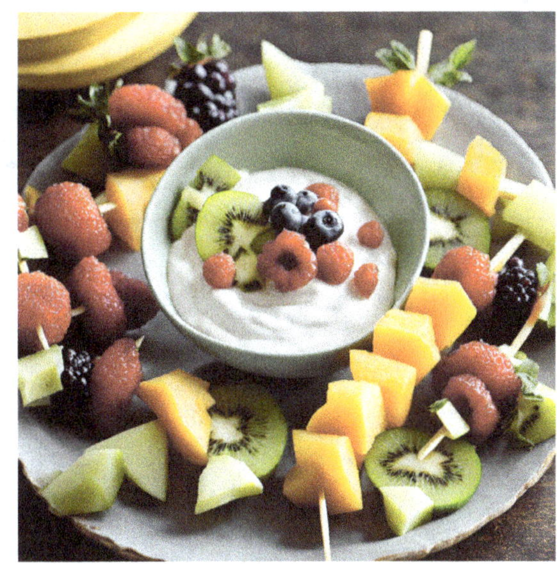

Preparation Time

Total: 15 minutes

Nutrition (per serving)

Calories: 100
Protein: 4g
Carbohydrates: 20g
Fiber: 3g
Fat: 1g

ingredients

For the Kabobs:

- 1 cup strawberries, hulled and halved
- 1 cup pineapple chunks
- 1 cup grapes
- 1 cup kiwi, peeled and sliced
- 1 cup blueberries

For the Yogurt Dip:

- 1 cup Greek yogurt
- 1 tablespoon honey
- 1 teaspoon vanilla extract

Instructions

1. Thread the fruit pieces onto wooden skewers, alternating the types of fruit for a colorful presentation.

2. Mix the Greek yoghurt, honey, and vanilla extract in a small bowl until well combined.

3. Serve the fruit kabobs with the yoghurt dip on the side.

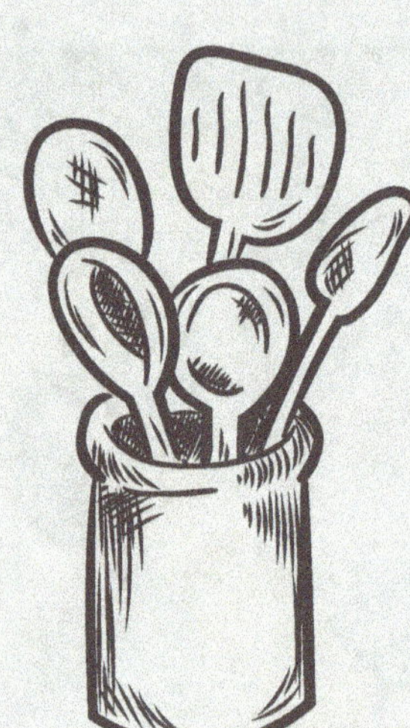

CHAPTER FIVE

★★★★★

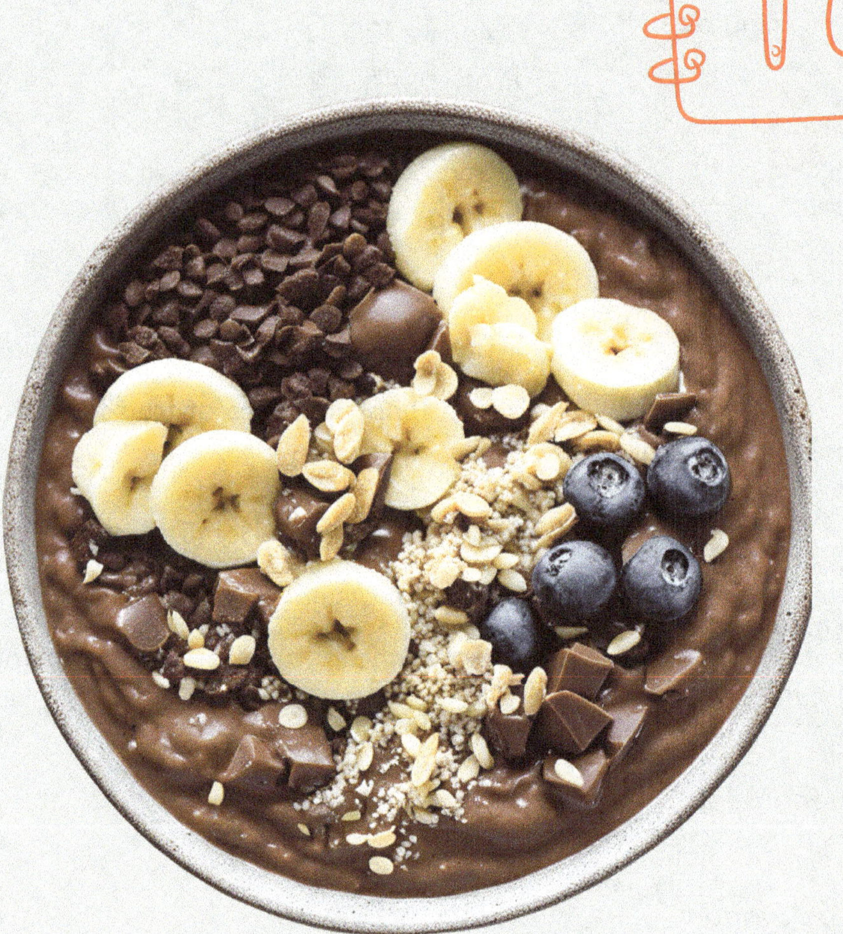

Snacks for Side Treats

About the recipe

Treat yourself to these refreshing and delicious Cottage Cheese and Pineapple Cups. This simple yet delightful combination of creamy cottage cheese and juicy pineapple makes for a perfect snack or light dessert that's both satisfying and healthy.

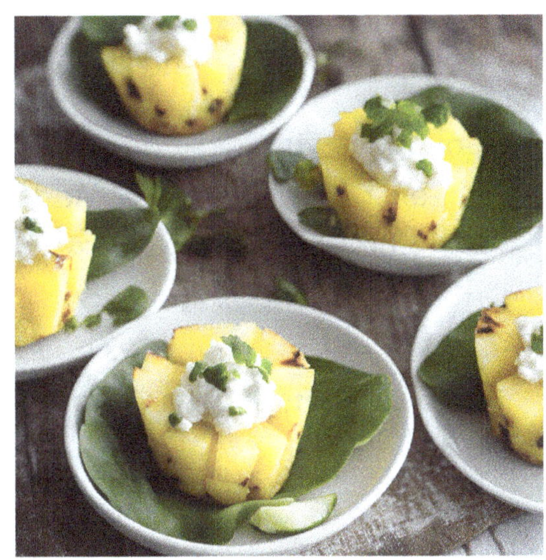

Cottage Cheese and Pineapple Cups

Preparation Time 

Total: 15 minutes

Nutrition (per serving)

Calories: 120
Protein: 10g
Carbohydrates: 15g
Fiber: 2g
Fat: 2g

ingredients

1 cup lowfat cottage cheese

1 cup pineapple chunks (fresh or canned, in juice)

1 tablespoon honey (optional)

A pinch of cinnamon (optional)

Instructions

1. Divide the cottage cheese evenly into two small bowls or cups.

2. Top each serving with pineapple chunks.

3. Drizzle with honey and sprinkle with cinnamon if desired.

4. Serve immediately and enjoy!

About the recipe

Cool down with these delightful Fruity Frozen Yogurt Popsicles. Made with fresh fruit and creamy Greek yoghurt, they are a refreshing and healthy treat perfect for hot days and fun to make with the whole family.

Fruity Frozen Yogurt Popsicles

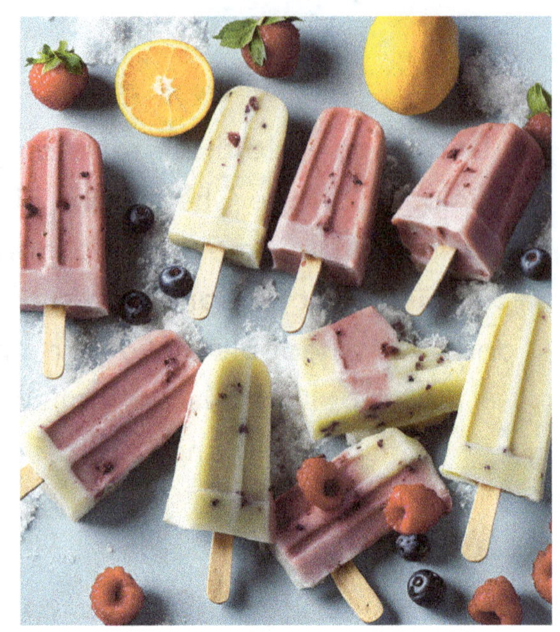

Preparation Time

4 hours and 10 minutes (including freezing time)

Nutrition (per serving)

Calories: 90
Protein: 6g
Carbohydrates: 15g
Fiber: 3g
Fat: 2g

ingredients

2 cups Greek yogurt
1 cup mixed berries (strawberries, blueberries, raspberries)
2 tablespoons honey
1 teaspoon vanilla extract

Instructions

1. Combine the Greek yoghurt, mixed berries, honey, and vanilla extract in a blender. Blend until smooth.

2. Pour the mixture into Popsicle molds.

3. Insert Popsicle sticks and freeze for at least 4 hours or until solid.

4. To remove the popsicles from the molds, run warm water over the outside of the molds for a few seconds.

5. Serve immediately and enjoy!

About the recipe

Start your day with these decadent yet healthy Chocolate Banana Smoothie Bowls. Packed with the goodness of bananas and rich cocoa, this smoothie bowl is a delightful breakfast or snack that feels indulgent but is entirely guilt free.

Chocolate Banana Smoothie Bowls

Preparation Time

Total: 10 minutes

Nutrition (per serving)

Calories: 150
Protein: 4g
Carbohydrates: 30g
Fiber: 6g
Fat: 3g

ingredients

2 frozen bananas
1 tablespoon unsweetened cocoa powder
1/2 cup almond milk (or any milk of choice)
1 tablespoon peanut butter (optional)
Toppings: sliced bananas, berries, granola, chia seeds

Instructions

1. In a blender, combine the frozen bananas, cocoa powder, almond milk, and peanut butter (if using). Blend until smooth and creamy.

2. Pour the smoothie into bowls.

3. Top with sliced bananas, berries, granola, and chia seeds.

4. Serve immediately and enjoy!

About the recipe

Enjoy a warm, comforting dessert with these Baked Apple Slices with Cinnamon. The natural sweetness of the apples combined with the spicy cinnamon makes for a delightful, healthy and satisfying treat.

Baked Apple Slices with Cinnamon

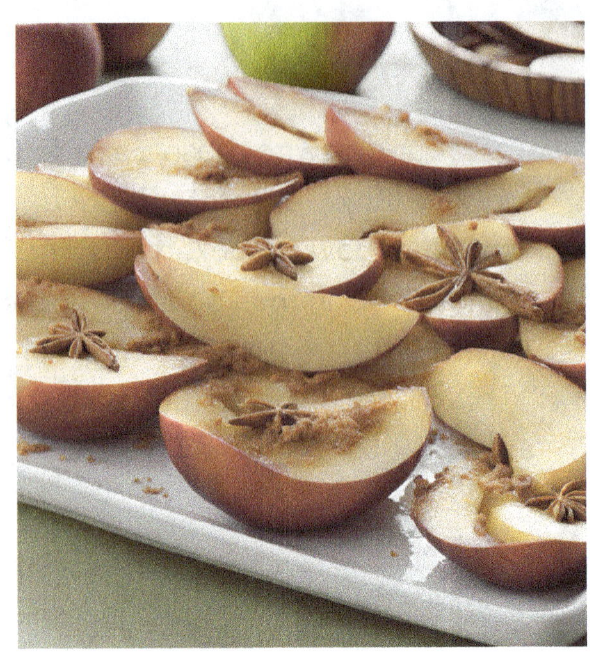

Preparation Time

Total: 30 minutes

Nutrition (per serving)

Calories: 100
Protein: 0g
Carbohydrates: 25g
Fiber: 5g
Fat: 0g

ingredients

4 apples, sliced

1 tablespoon cinnamon

1 tablespoon honey (optional)

Instructions

1. Preheat your oven to 375°F (190°C).

2. Arrange the apple slices on a baking sheet lined with parchment paper.

3. Sprinkle the apple slices with cinnamon and drizzle with honey if desired.

4. Bake for 2025 minutes until the apples are tender.

5. Serve warm and enjoy!

About the recipe

Indulge in a creamy, decadent treat with this Chocolate Avocado Mousse. Made with wholesome ingredients, it is rich in flavor and texture yet surprisingly healthy. It's the perfect dessert to satisfy your chocolate cravings.

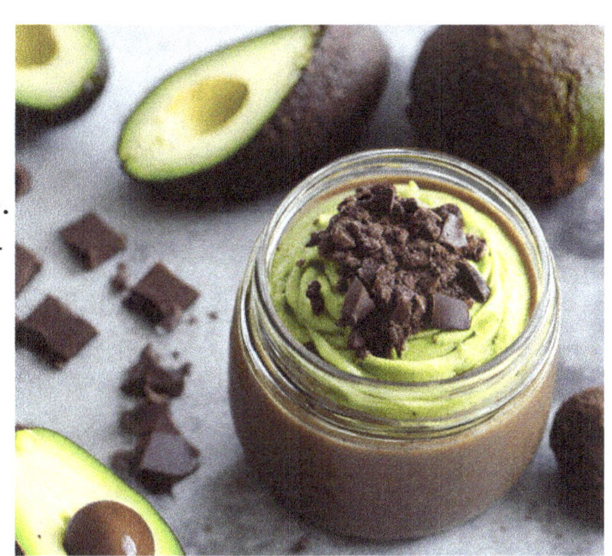

Chocolate Avocado Mousse

Preparation Time 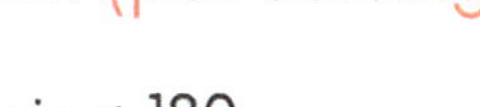

Total: 40 minutes (including refrigeration time)

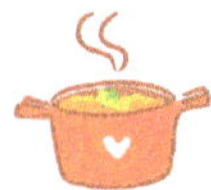

Nutrition (per serving)

Calories: 180
Protein: 2g
Carbohydrates: 20g
Fiber: 6g
Fat: 10g

ingredients

2 ripe avocados

1/4 cup unsweetened cocoa powder

1/4 cup honey

1 teaspoon vanilla extract

A pinch of sea salt

Instructions

1. In a food processor, blend the avocados until smooth.

2. Add the cocoa powder, honey, vanilla extract, and sea salt. Blend until well combined and creamy.

3. Spoon the mousse into small bowls or jars.

4. Refrigerate for at least 30 minutes before serving.

5. Serve chilled and enjoy!

About the recipe

These Crispy Baked Kale Chips are the perfect guilt free snack! They're super easy to make and packed with nutrients. Enjoy them as a snack or a crunchy addition to your meals.

Crispy Baked Kale Chips

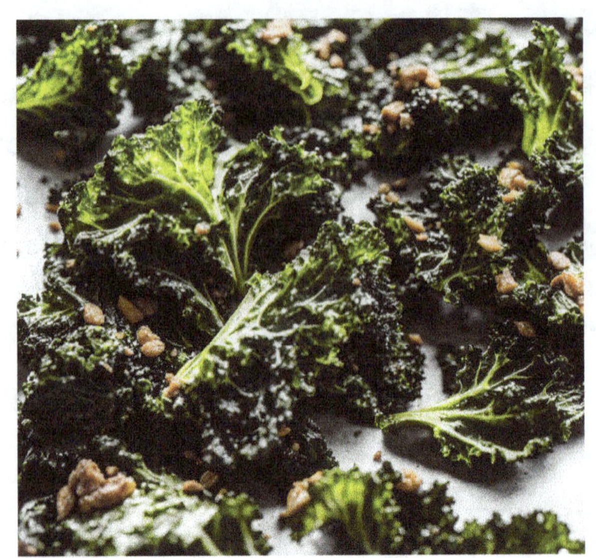

Preparation Time

Total: 20 minutes

Nutrition (per serving)

Nutrition (per serving):
Calories: 50
Protein: 2g
Carbohydrates: 7g
Fiber: 2g
Fat: 2g

ingredients

1 bunch of kale, washed and dried

1 tablespoon olive oil

1/2 teaspoon sea salt

Instructions

1. Preheat your oven to 350°F (175°C).

2. Remove the kale leaves from the stems and tear them into bite sized pieces.

3. Toss the kale with olive oil and sea salt in a large bowl.

4. Spread the kale leaves in a single layer on a baking sheet lined with parchment paper.

5. Bake for 1015 minutes until the edges are browned and crispy.

6. Let cool slightly before serving.

About the recipe

Enjoy a refreshing and satisfying snack with these Crunchy Carrot Sticks with Hummus. This combination perfectly balances crunch and creaminess, making it a delightful and healthy choice for any time of day.

Crunchy Carrot Sticks with Hummus

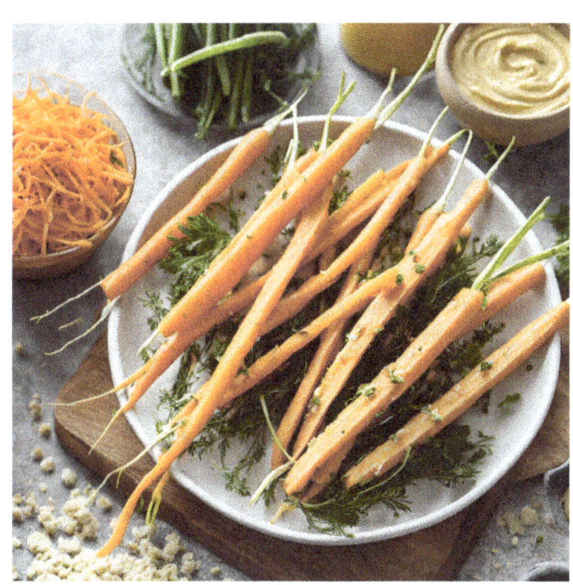

Preparation Time 

Total: 5 minutes

Nutrition (per serving)

Calories: 100
Protein: 4g
Carbohydrates: 15g
Fiber: 5g
Fat: 4g

ingredients

- 4 large carrots, peeled and cut into sticks
- 1 cup hummus (storebought or homemade)

Instructions

1. Peel the carrots and cut them into sticks.

2. Arrange the carrot sticks on a plate with a bowl of hummus.

3. Serve immediately, and enjoy dipping the carrots into the creamy hummus.

About the recipe

For a light and airy snack, try making Air Popped Popcorn. It's a classic treat that's delicious and incredibly low in calories. Perfect for movie nights or a quick bite!

Air Popped Popcorn

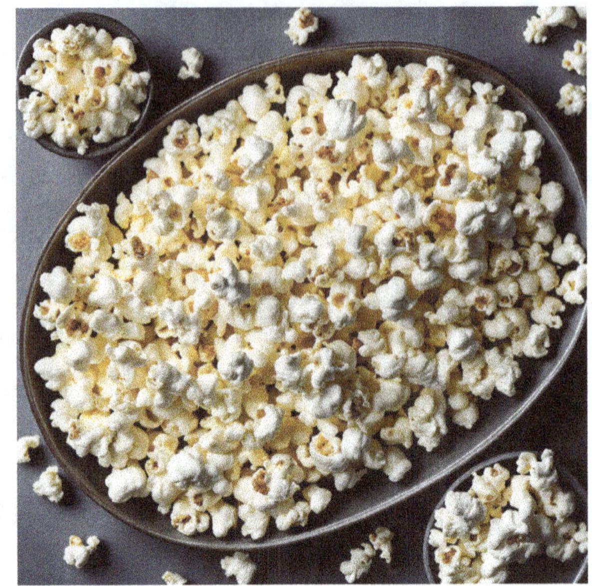

Preparation Time 

Total: 5 minutes

Nutrition (per serving)

Calories: 90
Protein: 3g
Carbohydrates: 18g
Fiber: 4g
Fat: 1g

ingredients

- 1/4 cup popcorn kernels
- Salt to taste

Instructions

1. Add the popcorn kernels to an air popper and follow the manufacturer's instructions to pop the kernels.

2. Transfer the popcorn to a large bowl and sprinkle with salt to taste.

3. Toss to combine and serve immediately.

About the recipe

Satisfy your sweet and savory cravings with Apple Slices with Peanut Butter. This quick, nutritious snack is perfect for a burst of energy anytime you need it.

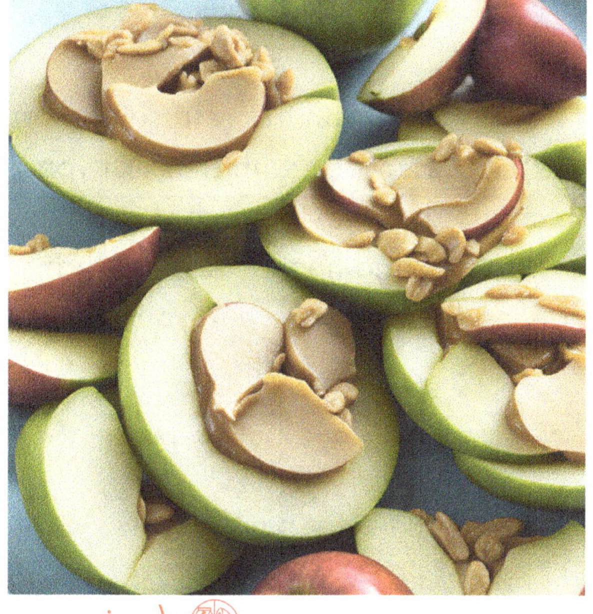

Apple Slices with Peanut Butter

Preparation Time 

Total: 5 minutes

Nutrition (per serving)

Calories: 150
Protein: 4g
Carbohydrates: 22g
Fiber: 4g
Fat: 7g

ingredients

- 1 large apple, sliced
- 2 tablespoons peanut butter (natural, no added sugar)

Instructions

1. Slice the apple into thin wedges.

2. Arrange the apple slices on a plate and serve with peanut butter for dipping.

3. Enjoy this delicious and nutritious snack!

About the recipe

Cool down with this refreshing Berry Sorbet. Made with a mix of your favorite berries, this sorbet is a sweet, tangy, and healthy dessert that's perfect for satisfying your sweet tooth.

Berry Sorbet

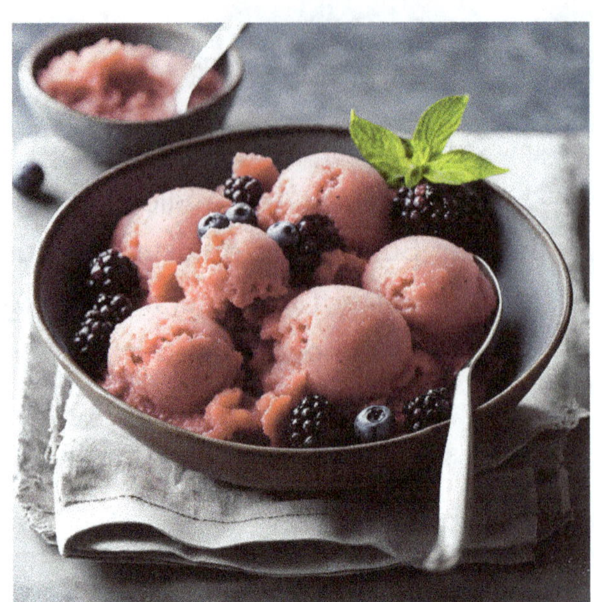

Preparation Time

Total: 2 hours (including freezing time)

Nutrition (per serving)

Calories: 80
Protein: 1g
Carbohydrates: 20g
Fiber: 6g
Fat: 0g

ingredients

- 2 cups mixed berries (strawberries, blueberries, raspberries)
- 1/4 cup water
- 1 tablespoon lemon juice
- 1 tablespoon honey (optional)

Instructions

1. Combine the mixed berries, water, lemon juice, and honey (if using) in a blender.
2. Blend until smooth.
3. Pour the mixture into a shallow container and freeze for 12 hours, stirring every 30 minutes until the sorbet is firm.
4. Scoop into bowls and serve immediately.

About the recipe

Enjoy the fresh and vibrant flavours of summer with this Minty Melon Salad. It's a light and refreshing dish that combines juicy melons with a hint of mint, perfect for an excellent and hydrating snack.

Minty Melon Salad

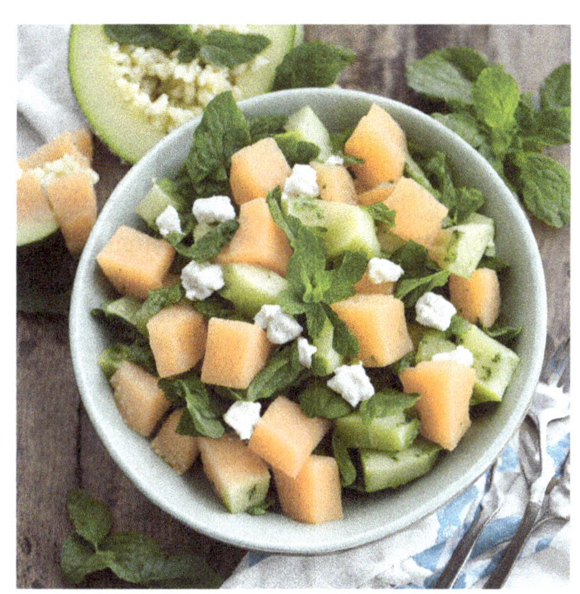

Preparation Time 

Total: 10 minutes

Nutrition (per serving)

Calories: 60
Protein: 1g
Carbohydrates: 15g
Fiber: 1g
Fat: 0g

ingredients

- 2 cups watermelon, cubed
- 2 cups cantaloupe, cubed
- 2 tablespoons fresh mint leaves, chopped
- 1 tablespoon lime juice

Instructions

1. In a large bowl, combine the watermelon and cantaloupe cubes.
2. Add the chopped mint leaves and lime juice.
3. Toss gently to combine.
4. Serve immediately or chill in the refrigerator until ready to serve.

About the recipe

This Kiwi Lime Sorbet is a tangy and refreshing treat perfect for a hot day. Combining kiwi and lime creates a delightful and refreshing dessert that's healthy and delicious.

Kiwi Lime Sorbet

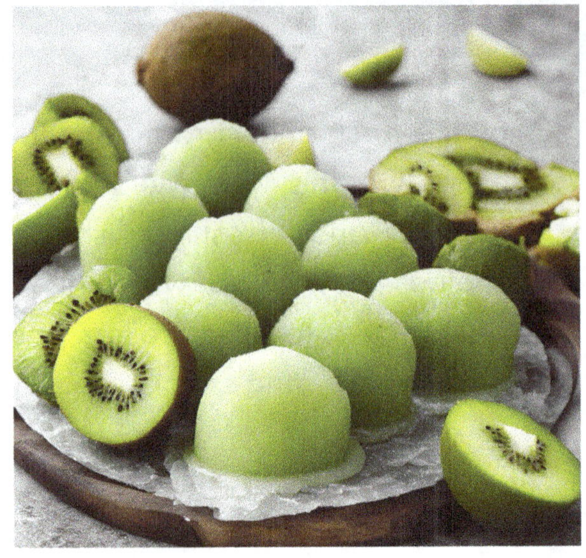

Preparation Time

Total: 2 hours (including freezing time)

Nutrition (per serving)

Calories: 70
Protein: 1g
Carbohydrates: 17g
Fiber: 3g

ingredients

- 4 ripe kiwis, peeled and chopped
- 1/4 cup lime juice
- 1 tablespoon honey (optional)

Instructions

1. Combine the chopped kiwis, lime juice, and honey (if using) in a blender.
2. Blend until smooth.
3. Pour the mixture into a shallow container and freeze for 12 hours, stirring every 30 minutes until the sorbet is firm.
4. Scoop into bowls and serve immediately.

One more favor

If you've enjoyed this book and found the recipes helpful, I would be grateful if you could leave a review. Your feedback helps other readers discover the benefits of healthy, delicious eating and supports the creation of more books like this one. Your thoughts and experiences are invaluable, and I would love to hear how these recipes have positively impacted your journey.

Happy cooking, and here's to a healthier, happier you!

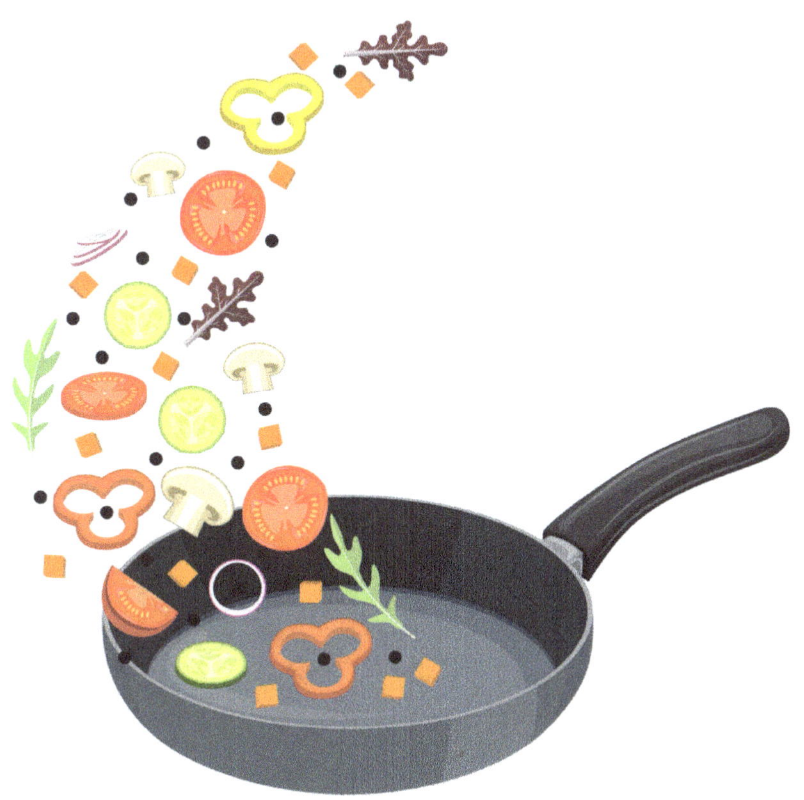

Conclusion

Congratulations on reaching the end of this collection of delightful, zero point weight loss recipes! You've embarked on a journey filled with vibrant flavors, nutritious ingredients, and exciting culinary adventures. Each recipe in this book was crafted with care to provide you with healthy, satisfying meals and snacks that won't derail your weight loss goals.

By now, you've likely discovered that eating healthily doesn't mean sacrificing taste or enjoyment. From the refreshing Minty Melon Salad to the indulgent Dark Chocolate Avocado Truffles, these recipes prove that delicious and nutritious can go hand in hand. Whether you're hosting a dinner party, preparing a quick weekday meal, or simply craving a guilt free treat, you now have various options.
Remember, consistency and balance is critical to successful weight loss and maintaining a healthy lifestyle. These recipes are designed to fit seamlessly into your daily routine, making it easier to stick to your goals without feeling deprived. Embrace the vibrant flavors, experiment with new ingredients, and enjoy creating wholesome meals that nourish your body and soul.

Thank you for allowing this book to be a part of your culinary journey. May it inspire you to continue exploring the world of healthy cooking, find joy in every bite, and achieve your weight loss goals with confidence and pleasure.

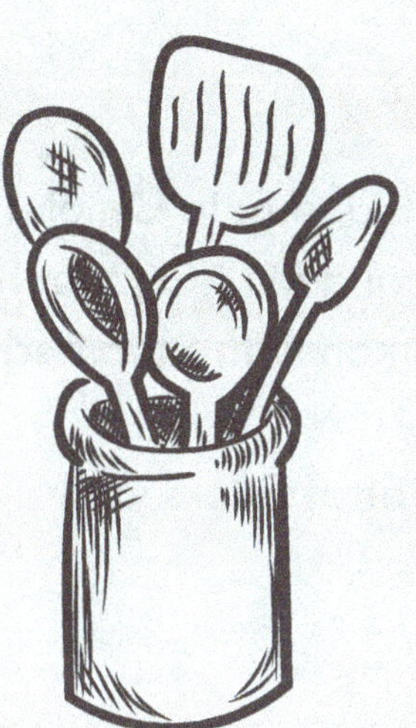

BONUS

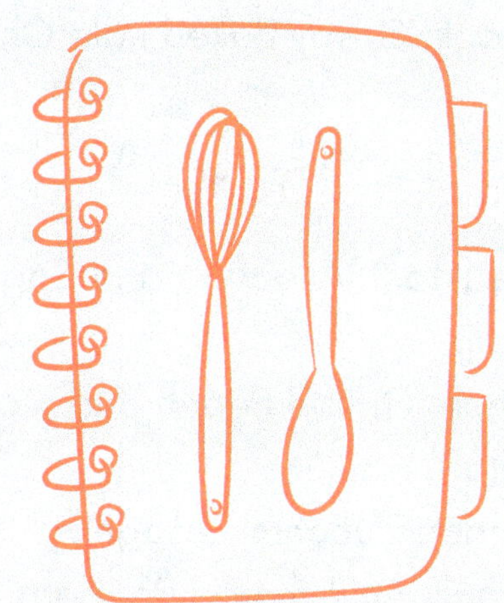

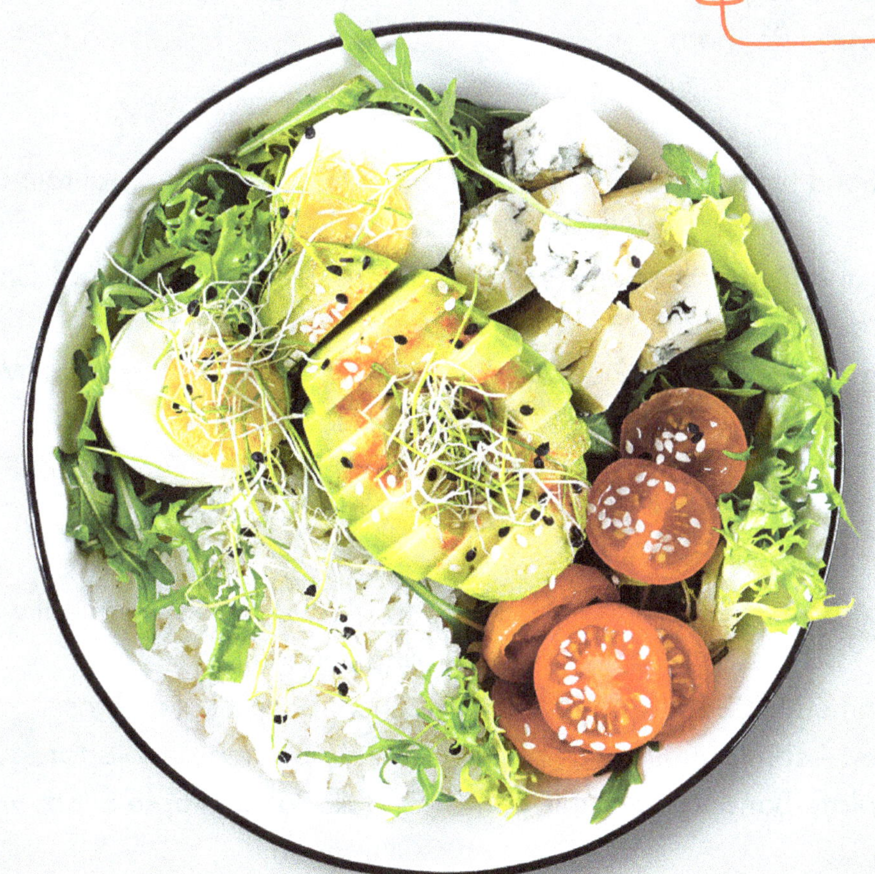

20 Days meal plan

DAY 1

Breakfast: Mixed Berry and Chia Smoothie
Lunch: Tomato Basil Soup
Dinner: Grilled Chicken with Quinoa and Avocado Salad
Snack: Crispy Baked Kale Chips

DAY 2

Breakfast: Spinach and Feta Omelet
Lunch: Cucumber and Mint Gazpacho
Dinner: Baked Salmon with Steamed Broccoli
Snack: Crunchy Carrot Sticks with Hummus

DAY 3

Breakfast: Avocado and Egg Breakfast Wrap
Lunch: Grilled Peach and Mozzarella Salad
Dinner: Zucchini Lasagna
Snack: Air-Popped Popcorn

DAY 4

Breakfast: Greek Yogurt with Honey and Walnuts
Lunch: Avocado and Grapefruit Salad
Dinner: Cauliflower Fried Rice
Snack: Apple Slices with Peanut Butter

DAY 5

Breakfast: Almond Flour Pancakes with Blueberries
Lunch: Carrot and Coriander Soup
Dinner: Vegetable and Bean Chili
Snack: Cottage Cheese and Pineapple Cups

DAY 6

Breakfast: Quinoa Breakfast Bowl with Mixed Fruit
Lunch: Beetroot and Goat Cheese Salad
Dinner: Turkey and Spinach Meatballs in Tomato Sauce
Snack: Fruity Frozen Yogurt Popsicles

DAY 7

Breakfast: Cottage Cheese and Peach Parfait
Lunch: Edamame with Sea Salt
Dinner: Stuffed Acorn Squash
Snack: Chocolate Banana Smoothie Bowls

DAY 8

Breakfast: Baked Oatmeal with Apples and Cinnamon
Lunch: Baked Kale Chips
Dinner: Shrimp and Asparagus Stir Fry
Snack: Baked Apple Slices with Cinnamon

DAY 9

Breakfast: Banana and Peanut Butter Toast
Lunch: Spicy Roasted Chickpeas
Dinner: Lentil and Sweet Potato Stew
Snack: Chocolate Avocado Mousse

DAY 10

Breakfast: Vegetable Frittata
Lunch: Zucchini Noodles with Pesto
Dinner: Eggplant Parmesan
Snack: Berry Sorbet

DAY 11

Breakfast: Tomato and Basil Bruschetta
Lunch: Stuffed Mini Bell Peppers
Dinner: Spaghetti Squash and Meatballs
Snack: Minty Melon Salad

DAY 12

Breakfast: Smoked Salmon and Avocado Bagel
Lunch: Watermelon and Feta Salad
Dinner: Grilled Portobello Mushrooms with Herbed Quinoa
Snack: Kiwi Lime Sorbet

DAY 13

Breakfast: Overnight Oats with Raspberry and Chia
Lunch: Caprese Skewers with Balsamic Glaze
Dinner: Chicken Fajitas with Bell Peppers and Onion
Snack: Cottage Cheese and Pineapple Cups

DAY 14

Breakfast: Mushroom and Spinach Scrambled Eggs
Lunch: Roasted Brussel Sprouts with Garlic
Dinner: Baked Cod with Ratatouille
Snack: Berry Sorbet

DAY 15

Breakfast: Whole Grain Waffles with Fresh Strawberries
Lunch: Cauliflower Buffalo Bites
Dinner: Veggie Burger with Sweet Potato Bun
Snack: Chocolate Avocado Mousse

DAY 16

Breakfast: Poached Eggs over Asparagus Spears
Lunch: Broccoli and Almond Soup
Dinner: Butternut Squash Soup with a Twist of Ginger
Snack: Minty Melon Salad

DAY 17

Breakfast: Sweet Potato and Black Bean
Breakfast Burrito
Lunch: Arugula and Parmesan Salad
Dinner: Quinoa Salad with Roasted
Vegetables
Snack: Apple Slices with Peanut Butter

DAY 18

Breakfast: Zucchini and Carrot Muffins
Lunch: Sweet Potato Fries with
Avocado Dip
Dinner: Stuffed Peppers with Ground
Turkey and Quinoa
Snack: Cottage Cheese and Pineapple
Cups

DAY 19

Breakfast: Breakfast Quinoa with Almond
Milk
Lunch: Greek Salad with Lemon Dressing
Dinner: Pan-Seared Tuna with Avocado
Salsa
Snack: Fruity Frozen Yogurt Popsicles

DAY 20

Breakfast: Baked Peaches with
Almond Crumble
Lunch: Spinach and Artichoke Dip
Dinner: Roasted Vegetable and
Hummus Wraps
Snack: Chocolate Banana Smoothie
Bowls

Happy Cooking !!!